THE NOURISHII LOW-FODMAP DIET COOKBOOK

Relieve IBS, Eliminate Bloat, and Restore Your Digestive Health with Delicious Recipes and a 60-Day Meal Plan

Serena Willow

Table of Contents

❧ HERE IS YOUR FREE GIFTS! ❧

SCAN HERE TO DOWNLOAD

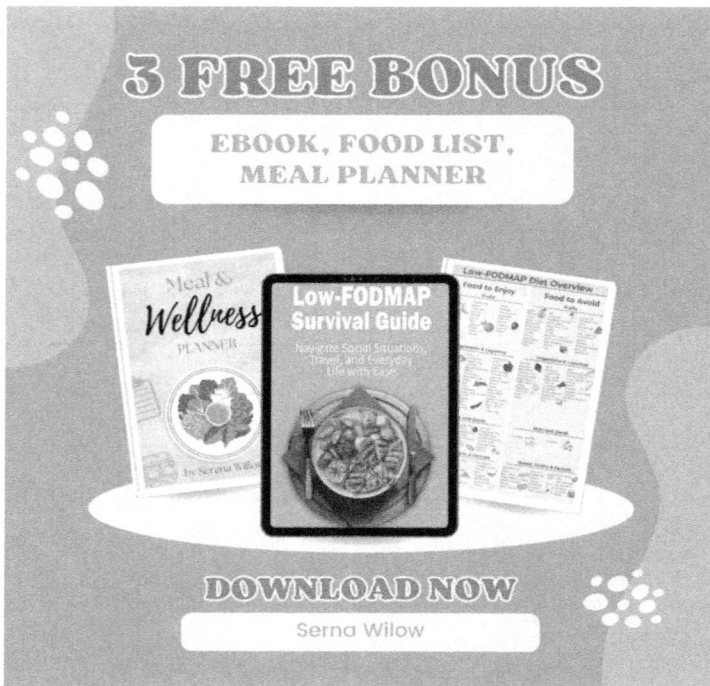

3 FREE BONUS

EBOOK, FOOD LIST, MEAL PLANNER

DOWNLOAD NOW

Serna Wilow

In this extra content you'll get:

1. Essential Low-FODMAP Food List
A comprehensive list of foods to eat and avoid for optimal digestive health.

2. Low-FODMAP Survival Guide
Navigate social situations, eat on the go, and maintain your Low-FODMAP lifestyle with ease.

3. Ultimate Meal & Wellness Planner
Keep your Low-FODMAP journey organized with diet guidelines, recipes, and lifestyle tips at your fingertips.

SCAN HERE TO DOWNLOAD IT

Introduction

Embarking on the journey to better digestive health can feel overwhelming—especially for those dealing with Irritable Bowel Syndrome (IBS) or chronic digestive discomfort. This cookbook is designed to be a beacon of clarity and relief, guiding you through the transformative power of the Low-FODMAP diet—a scientifically backed approach proven to ease symptoms by targeting specific fermentable carbohydrates known as FODMAPs.

For many, the term FODMAP is unfamiliar. These fermentable sugars—Oligosaccharides, Disaccharides, Monosaccharides, and Polyols—are found in everyday foods like apples, wheat, milk, and onions. For individuals with IBS, they can cause bloating, pain, and digestive irregularity. This book simplifies the science, helping you understand which foods to avoid and which to embrace for a calmer gut and a more comfortable life.

But this isn't just about what you can't eat—it's about discovering what you can. With 120 carefully crafted recipes for breakfasts, lunches, dinners, snacks, and desserts, this cookbook proves that dietary management and culinary enjoyment can go hand in hand. Each recipe is easy to follow, even for beginners, making it simple to prepare nourishing meals without stress.

Beyond the recipes, this guide provides essential tools to support you throughout every phase of your Low-FODMAP journey—from elimination to reintroduction. It offers clear strategies for tracking symptoms, identifying trigger foods, and personalizing your diet in a sustainable way.

Importantly, this book also addresses the emotional side of living with IBS—the frustration of unpredictable symptoms, the anxiety around social events, and the fear that food has become an enemy. Through practical advice and encouraging guidance, it helps you reclaim a sense of control and joy in your relationship with food.

The Nourishing Low-FODMAP Diet Cookbook isn't just a collection of recipes—it's a complete roadmap for regaining your health and quality of life. Whether you're newly diagnosed or seeking better ways to manage your symptoms, this book offers not just information, but hope..

Welcome to Your Low-FODMAP Journey

Starting your Low-FODMAP journey opens the door to a transformative path toward better digestive health and a higher quality of life. This diet, focused on reducing intake of certain fermentable carbs, offers a promising solution for those plagued by IBS and related digestive issues.

While the concept may seem daunting at first, the goal of this guide is to simplify the process, making it accessible and manageable for everyone, regardless of their culinary expertise or nutritional knowledge. By carefully selecting ingredients that minimize digestive distress, you can create meals that are not only nourishing but also delicious and satisfying.

This journey is not about restriction but about discovering new foods and flavors that enhance your well-being. As you turn these pages, you'll find yourself equipped with the tools and confidence needed to navigate this diet successfully, leading to a happier, healthier you.

The Significance of Gut Health

Gut health is foundational to our overall well-being, influencing not just digestion but also the immune system, mental health, and risk of chronic diseases. The digestive system is more than a food processing plant; it's a complex ecosystem where nutrients are absorbed, and waste is expelled.

An imbalance in this system can cause pain, inflammation, and a variety of digestive diseases, such as Irritable Bowel Syndrome (IBS). A robust immune system, heart health, brain health, better mood, good sleep, efficient digestion, and possibly even the prevention of some malignancies and autoimmune illnesses are all influenced by a healthy gut.

An important variable in this is the equilibrium between good and bad bacteria in the gut microbiome. Diets high in processed foods and sugar can disrupt this balance, leading to increased "bad" bacteria, which can trigger inflammation and increase the risk of disease.

Embracing a Low-FODMAP diet can help restore this balance by eliminating foods that are difficult to digest and that feed harmful bacteria, promoting a healthier gut microbiome. This, in turn, can lead to significant improvements in digestive health and overall quality of life, making understanding and caring for your gut an essential part of maintaining good health.

What are FODMAPs

FODMAPs stand for Fermentable Oligo-, Di-, Mono-saccharides And Polyols, a group of small-chain carbohydrates that are poorly absorbed in the small intestine. These sugars are fermented by bacteria in the large intestine, where they take in water and produce gas. Symptoms including gas, bloating, diarrhea, constipation, and stomach pain can result from this process, especially in those who have Irritable Bowel Syndrome (IBS).

Several fruits, vegetables, dairy products, cereals, and sweeteners are common sources of fructooligosaccharides (FODMAPS). Reducing the consumption of these fermentable carbohydrates is the goal of the Low-FODMAP diet, which can help people who are having digestive problems. Through the identification and restriction of foods rich in FODMAPs, people can enhance their quality of life and digestive health by effectively managing their symptoms. Given that individual tolerance to fructooligosaccharides (FODMAPS) can vary widely, this dietary approach highlights the significance of customization.

Definition and Types of FODMAPs

FODMAPs are a collection of short-chain carbohydrates that are not well absorbed in the gut, leading to symptoms in people with sensitive digestive systems, such as those with IBS. These include:

Fermentable Oligosaccharides: found in foods like wheat, rye, legumes, and various fruits and vegetables.

Disaccharides: notably lactose from dairy products.

Monosaccharides: exemplified by fructose in certain fruits, honey, and agave nectar.

Polyols: sugar alcohols that are present in certain fruits, vegetables, and artificial sweeteners.

Each type of FODMAP can contribute to the common symptoms of digestive discomfort, including bloating, gas, and abdominal pain. By understanding these categories and their food sources, individuals can tailor their diets to minimize intake of high-FODMAP foods, potentially alleviating IBS symptoms. This approach allows for a personalized dietary plan that focuses on reducing the fermentable sugars responsible for gastrointestinal distress.

How FODMAPs Affect Digestion and IBS

FODMAPs, when ingested by individuals with IBS, can lead to increased water in the intestine and excessive gas production as they are fermented by gut bacteria. This process often results in significant discomfort, manifesting as bloating, abdominal pain, and altered bowel habits such as constipation and diarrhea. The sensitivity to these symptoms varies widely among individuals, making the management of IBS a highly personalized journey.

The Low-FODMAP diet, by limiting the intake of these fermentable sugars, aims to reduce the osmotic effect and fermentation in the large intestine, thereby alleviating the distressing gastrointestinal symptoms. This dietary strategy not only helps in identifying specific triggers but also in understanding the intricate relationship between diet and digestive health.

By adopting a Low-FODMAP diet, individuals can effectively manage their IBS symptoms, leading to improved digestive function and overall quality of life.

Research and Evidence Supporting the Diet

The Low-FODMAP diet, developed by researchers at Monash University in Australia, is backed by extensive scientific research. Numerous studies have demonstrated its effectiveness in reducing symptoms of Irritable Bowel Syndrome (IBS) and improving the quality of life for individuals with functional gastrointestinal disorders.

A study published in "Gastroenterology" in 2014 by Halmos et al. found that IBS patients following a Low-FODMAP diet experienced significant reductions in symptoms like bloating, abdominal pain, and altered bowel habits compared to those on a standard diet. Another study in "Clinical Gastroenterology and Hepatology" in 2016 by Staudacher et al. confirmed these findings, with approximately 75% of IBS patients reporting symptom relief on a Low-FODMAP diet.

Moreover, research published in "Alimentary Pharmacology & Therapeutics" has shown that the Low-FODMAP diet not only alleviates IBS symptoms but also positively impacts gut microbiota. The study found a reduction in gas-producing bacteria, which are often responsible for bloating and discomfort.

The efficacy of the Low-FODMAP diet is further supported by randomized controlled trials and systematic reviews, establishing it as a first-line dietary intervention for managing IBS. These studies underscore the diet's ability to provide sustained symptom relief and enhance the overall well-being of individuals suffering from IBS.

Intro to Low-FODMAP Diet

Embarking on the Low-FODMAP diet begins with identifying and eliminating high-FODMAP foods from your diet, which are known to trigger digestive discomfort. This initial phase, known as the elimination phase, is crucial for setting the foundation of your journey towards better digestive health.

Start by familiarizing yourself with common high-FODMAP ingredients such as garlic, onions, wheat, and certain dairy products, and begin substituting these with low-FODMAP alternatives like green onions (green parts only), gluten-free grains, and lactose-free dairy. It's also essential to read food labels carefully, as many processed foods contain hidden FODMAPs.

Planning your meals and preparing food at home can significantly help in managing your intake and avoiding accidental consumption of high-FODMAP foods. Remember, the goal is not to restrict your diet indefinitely but to identify your personal triggers and create a balanced, enjoyable eating plan that supports your digestive health.

The Elimination Phase

The Elimination Phase is the initial, critical step in the Low-FODMAP journey, focusing on removing high-FODMAP foods from your diet for a period of 4-6 weeks. This stage is designed to give your digestive system a break and to identify which foods might be causing your symptoms.

During this time, it's vital to eliminate all foods known to be high in FODMAPs, including certain fruits, vegetables, grains, dairy products, and sweeteners. This doesn't mean your diet will lack variety or flavor; instead, you'll explore a new world of low-FODMAP alternatives that are just as satisfying and delicious.

Keeping a detailed food diary during this phase is crucial. It helps track what you eat and how it affects your symptoms, providing invaluable insights for the next stage of the diet.

Patience and commitment are key, as it takes time for your body to adjust and for symptoms to improve. Remember, this phase is temporary, setting the stage for a more personalized and flexible approach to managing your digestive health in the long term.

Sample 7-Day Meal Plan for the Elimination Phase

DAY 1

- **Breakfast:** Blueberry Almond Overnight Oats

✓ Ingredients: Gluten-free oats, almond milk, chia seeds, blueberries, and a touch of maple syrup.

- **Lunch:** Grilled Chicken Caesar Salad

✓ Ingredients: Romaine lettuce, grilled chicken breast, lactose-free Parmesan cheese, homemade Low-FODMAP Caesar dressing.

- **Dinner:** Lemon Herb Chicken Thighs with Roasted Carrots

✓ Ingredients: Chicken thighs, lemon juice, olive oil, fresh herbs (like rosemary and thyme), and roasted carrots.

Snack: Rice Cakes with Peanut Butter

✓ Ingredients: Plain rice cakes, natural peanut butter.

DAY 2

- **Breakfast:** Banana Walnut Pancakes

✓ Ingredients: Gluten-free flour, almond milk, ripe banana, walnuts, and eggs.

- **Lunch:** Quinoa and Roasted Vegetable Bowl

✓ Ingredients: Quinoa, roasted bell peppers, zucchini, and carrots with a drizzle of olive oil.

- **Dinner:** Baked Salmon with Lemon Dill Sauce and Steamed Carrots

✓ Ingredients: Salmon fillet, lemon juice, fresh dill, olive oil, and carrots.

- **Snack:** Lactose-Free Greek Yogurt with Strawberries

✓ Ingredients: Lactose-free Greek yogurt, fresh strawberries.

DAY 3

- **Breakfast:** Spinach and Feta Omelette

✓ Ingredients: Eggs, fresh spinach, lactose-free feta cheese, and olive oil.

- **Lunch:** Turkey and Swiss Sandwich on Gluten-Free Bread

✓ Ingredients: Gluten-free bread, turkey slices, Swiss cheese, lettuce, and tomato.

- **Dinner:** Citrus Herb Grilled Chicken with Brown Rice

✓ Ingredients: Chicken breast, lemon juice, olive oil, fresh herbs, and brown rice.

- **Snack:** Carrot and Cucumber Sticks with Zucchini Hummus

✓ Ingredients: Carrot sticks, cucumber sticks, Low-FODMAP hummus.

DAY 4

- **Breakfast:** Sweet Potato Hash with Eggs

✓ Ingredients: Sweet potato, eggs, bell pepper, and olive oil.

- **Lunch:** Chicken and Mixed Greens Salad

✓ Ingredients: Grilled chicken, mixed greens, Low-FODMAP dressing.

- **Dinner:** Baked Cod with Dill and Roasted Potatoes

✓ Ingredients: Cod fillet, fresh dill, olive oil, lemon juice, and baby potatoes.

- **Snack:** Popcorn with a sprinkle of sea salt

✓ Ingredients: Popcorn kernels, olive oil, sea salt.

DAY 5

- **Breakfast:** Greek Yogurt Parfait

✓ Ingredients: Lactose-free Greek yogurt, gluten-free granola, fresh blueberries.

- **Lunch:** Tuna Salad Lettuce Wraps

✓ Ingredients: Tuna in water, mayonnaise (Low-FODMAP), lettuce leaves, and diced cucumber.

- **Dinner:** Beef and Bell Pepper Stir-Fry

✓ Ingredients: Lean beef strips, bell peppers, soy sauce (Low-FODMAP), and ginger.

- **Snack:** Almonds and a small banana

✓ Ingredients: Almonds, banana (small and ripe).

DAY 6

- **Breakfast:** Chia Seed Pudding with Berries

✓ Ingredients: Chia seeds, almond milk, fresh berries, and a touch of maple syrup.

- **Lunch:** Mediterranean Veggie Salad

✓ Ingredients: Cucumber, cherry tomatoes, red bell pepper, zucchini, green onion tops, Kalamata olives, lactose-free feta cheese, fresh herbs (parsley & mint), lemon juice, and olive oil.

- **Dinner:** Lemon Shrimp Skewers with Quinoa

✓ Ingredients: Shrimp, lemon juice, olive oil, fresh herbs, and quinoa.

- **Snack:** Rice Paper Veggie Rolls

✓ Ingredients: Rice paper, carrots, cucumbers, lettuce, and a Low-FODMAP dipping sauce.

DAY 7

- **Breakfast:** Buckwheat Porridge

✓ Ingredients: Buckwheat groats, almond milk, cinnamon, and a drizzle of maple syrup.

- **Lunch:** Mediterranean Quinoa Bowl

✓ Ingredients: Quinoa, diced cucumber, cherry tomatoes, red bell peppers, parsley, lemon juice, olive oil, salt, and pepper.

- **Dinner:** Grilled Mahi Mahi with Pineapple Salsa

✓ Ingredients: Mahi Mahi fillets, pineapple, red bell pepper, lime juice, and cilantro.

- **Snack:** Cottage Cheese and Pineapple Bowl

✓ Ingredients: Lactose-free cottage cheese, fresh pineapple chunks.

Monitor Your Symptoms: Keep a food and symptom diary to track how your body responds to each meal.

Stay Hydrated: Drink plenty of water throughout the day to support digestion and overall health.

Avoid Large Portions: Stick to recommended portion sizes to prevent overloading your digestive system.

Consult with a Professional: If you have any concerns or need personalized advice, consider consulting with a dietitian or healthcare provider.

This 7-day meal plan is designed to provide a balanced and varied diet while strictly adhering to the Low-FODMAP guidelines, helping you manage your IBS symptoms effectively.

The Reintroduction Phase

The Reintroduction Phase is a pivotal moment in your Low-FODMAP journey, where you gradually reintroduce high-FODMAP foods back into your diet to pinpoint your personal triggers. This stage requires careful planning and observation.

Start by introducing one food from a single FODMAP group at a time, in small amounts, and monitor your symptoms over three days. If a particular food causes discomfort, you know it's a trigger and should be limited or avoided in your diet. Conversely, if there's no adverse effect, you can safely incorporate it into your meals.

This methodical process not only helps in identifying specific foods that exacerbate your symptoms but also expands your dietary options, making your meals more varied and enjoyable.

It's essential to keep a detailed food and symptom diary during this phase, noting the type of food, the amount consumed, and any symptoms experienced. This personalized approach empowers you to create a balanced, sustainable diet tailored to your digestive system's needs, ultimately leading to improved gut health and a better quality of life. Remember, patience and attentiveness are key during this phase as you learn more about your body's responses to different foods.

Long-Term Management of IBS

Managing IBS effectively over the long term requires a balanced approach that goes beyond the initial phases of the Low-FODMAP diet. After identifying personal triggers, the focus shifts to integrating a wide variety of low-FODMAP foods to ensure nutritional balance and variety in your diet. Regular monitoring of symptoms is crucial, as tolerance levels to different foods may change over time. Incorporating stress-reduction techniques such as yoga, meditation, or regular exercise can also play a significant role in managing IBS symptoms, as stress is a known trigger.

Staying informed about new research and dietary recommendations can provide additional strategies for symptom management. Creating a community of support with friends, family, medical experts, and/or online forums can provide guidance and encouragement.

Remember, managing IBS is a personal journey that requires patience, experimentation, and resilience. With the right strategies, it is possible to live a full and active life despite IBS.

Tailoring the Diet to Your Needs

The Low-FODMAP diet is not a one-size-fits-all solution; it requires careful personalization to meet individual needs and preferences. After completing the elimination and reintroduction phases, you will have a clearer understanding of which foods trigger your symptoms and which ones you can tolerate. Tailoring the diet to your needs involves continuously adjusting your food choices based on your body's responses.

First, maintain a detailed food and symptom diary. This ongoing record helps identify patterns and potential triggers that may not have been apparent during the initial phases. It's essential to note not only what you eat but also the quantities and any symptoms experienced. This meticulous tracking allows for fine-tuning your diet to enhance comfort and well-being.

Second, embrace flexibility and variety within the low-FODMAP framework. Try a variety of low-FODMAP foods and recipes to avoid diet boredom and make sure you're getting enough nutrients. Including a variety of cereals, fruits, vegetables, proteins, and other foods keeps the nutritional balance intact and promotes general health.

Third, consider consulting with a dietitian experienced in the Low-FODMAP diet. A professional can provide personalized advice, suggest alternative foods, and help develop strategies to manage social and dining-out situations. This guidance ensures that your diet remains both effective and enjoyable.

Finally, stay informed about the latest research and developments in digestive health. New findings can offer insights into additional foods or practices that may benefit you.

By continuously adapting and personalizing the Low-FODMAP diet, you can manage your IBS symptoms effectively while enjoying a varied and satisfying diet that caters to your unique needs.

Maintaining Nutritional Balance

Maintaining nutritional balance on a Low-FODMAP diet involves careful planning to ensure you're getting a wide array of nutrients while adhering to dietary restrictions. It's crucial to incorporate a variety of low-FODMAP fruits, vegetables, grains, proteins, and fats into your meals to cover all nutritional bases.

Paying attention to portion sizes helps manage IBS symptoms while also meeting your body's needs for vitamins, minerals, and other essential nutrients. Diversifying your diet not only prevents nutritional deficiencies but also makes meals more enjoyable and satisfying.

Consider consulting with a dietitian who can provide personalized advice and help you design a balanced meal plan that accommodates your dietary restrictions and health goals. By doing so, you can support your digestive health and overall well-being without compromising on taste or nutrition.

Shopping list

Crafting a shopping list tailored to the Low-FODMAP diet is a pivotal step in managing IBS symptoms effectively. This list is designed to simplify your grocery shopping, ensuring you have all the necessary ingredients to prepare the delicious and nutritious recipes found in this cookbook. Embrace this list as a tool to navigate the grocery aisles with confidence, selecting foods that support your digestive health.

Fruits and Vegetables: Opt for Low-FODMAP fruits like strawberries, oranges, blueberries, pineapple, cantaloupe, kiwi. Include a variety of vegetables such as carrots, spinach, and bell peppers. Remember, portion sizes are key to keeping these options low-FODMAP.

Proteins: Stock up on lean meats like chicken breast, lean beef, turkey, and pork loin. Include eggs and plant-based proteins such as firm tofu, tempeh and canned lentils (in small amounts), ensuring they are rinsed well before use.

Dairy and Dairy Alternatives: Choose lactose-free milk, yogurt, and cheese. Almond milk and coconut yogurt are great dairy-free options that are Low-FODMAP friendly.

Grains: Look for gluten-free pasta, bread, and oatmeal. Quinoa and brown rice are excellent choices for adding variety to your meals.

Nuts and Seeds: Almonds, walnuts, peanuts, macadamias, chia seeds are good options in moderation. Keep servings to a handful to maintain Low-FODMAP compliance.

Oils and Fats: Olive oil and garlic-infused oil are great for cooking and dressings. Avoid high-FODMAP oils like coconut oil in large quantities.

Seasonings: Fresh herbs, salt, pepper, and most non-onion, non-garlic spices can add flavor to your recipes without adding FODMAPs.

Snacks: Look for gluten-free and Low-FODMAP certified snacks for convenience. Rice cakes, lactose-free cheese, and small servings of nuts can be good options.

Beverages: Stick to water, lactose-free milk, and non-caffeinated herbal teas. Avoid high-FODMAP choices like apple juice and soft drinks with high fructose corn syrup.

Keep in mind that diversity and moderation are essential for a low-FODMAP diet to be successful. This shopping list should be used as a reference, but you should constantly be aware of how your body reacts to different foods and make any adjustments. Cheers to a healthy and delicious shopping experience while following the Low-FODMAP diet.

★★★★★

I put a lot of effort into writing this book, so after you've completed, I would really appreciate it if you could give it an Amazon review. It would make possible the distribution of this information.

Low-FODMAP Recipes

The recipes in this chapter are designed to help you enjoy flavorful meals while managing IBS symptoms. Some ingredients used—though not strictly low-FODMAP—are included in controlled portions that many individuals tolerate well. For instance, broccoli heads are lower in FODMAPs than the stems and can be consumed in moderate amounts. Likewise, avocados may be acceptable in servings of 30g or less.

Your experience may differ, so listen to your body and adjust the recipes to suit your personal digestive response. The ultimate goal is a diverse, enjoyable diet that supports your well-being.

Important Note on Ingredients and FODMAP Tolerances

After completing the Elimination Phase, certain foods can often be reintroduced gradually and safely in specific portion sizes. Ingredients such as avocado, almonds, lentils, chickpeas, black beans, green beans, and dairy products (like aged cheese or lactose-free milk) may be tolerated by some individuals—but only in limited, Monash-approved quantities. When such ingredients appear in recipes, their low-FODMAP serving sizes have been clearly noted.

This flexibility allows you to broaden your food choices while staying symptom-free. However, always proceed with caution and consult a qualified dietitian if you're unsure. What works for one person might not work for another—and that's perfectly normal.

Breakfasts

1. Blueberry Almond Overnight Oats

Prep time: 8 hours (overnight soaking)

Cook time: 0 minutes

Serves: 2

Ingredients:

- 1 cup gluten-free rolled oats

- 1 ½ cups almond milk, unsweetened

- ¼ cup blueberries, fresh or frozen

- 2 tablespoons almond butter

- 1 tablespoon chia seeds

- 1 tablespoon maple syrup (optional)

- ½ teaspoon vanilla extract

- Pinch of salt

- Sliced almonds, for garnish

Preparation instructions:

1. Mix together the rolled oats, almond milk, chia seeds, vanilla extract, maple syrup (if using), and a small pinch of salt in a medium-sized mixing bowl. Stir well to mix.

2. Take care not to crush the blueberries as you gently fold them in.

3. Divide the mixture evenly between two jars or containers with lids. Seal the containers and refrigerate overnight, or for at least 8 hours.

4. Before serving, stir the oats well. To get the right consistency, thin out any extra mixture by adding a little amount of almond milk.

5. Garnish with sliced almonds and additional blueberries on top.

Per serving: Calories: 345; Fat: 14g; Protein: 10g; Carbs: 46g; Sugar: 10g (without optional maple syrup); Fiber: 9g

Difficulty rating: ★☆☆☆☆

Allergen information: Contains nuts (almonds). Gluten-free.

---

2. Spinach and Feta Omelette

Prep time: 10 minutes

Cook time: 5 minutes

Serves: 2

Ingredients:

- 4 large eggs

- 2 tablespoons lactose-free milk

- 1/2 cup fresh spinach, chopped

- 1/4 cup feta cheese, crumbled

- 1 tablespoon olive oil

- Salt and pepper, to taste

Preparation instructions:

1. Beat the eggs, lactose-free milk, salt, and pepper in a medium-sized bowl until thoroughly mixed.

2. In a nonstick skillet, warm the olive oil over medium heat.

3. Add the chopped spinach to the skillet and sauté for 1-2 minutes, or until slightly wilted.

4. Cover the spinach with the egg mixture. Cook for two to three minutes, or until the edges of the eggs start to set.

5. Sprinkle the crumbled feta cheese over half of the omelette. Gently fold the remaining omelette half over the cheese using a spatula.

6. Continue to cook for another 1-2 minutes, or until the cheese is melted and the eggs are fully set.

7. Carefully slide the omelette onto a plate and serve immediately.

Per serving: Calories: 290; Fat: 22g; Protein: 19g; Carbs: 3g; Sugar: 2g; Fiber: 0.5g

Difficulty rating: ★☆☆☆☆

---

3. Banana Walnut Pancakes

Prep time: 10 minutes

Cook time: 15 minutes

Serves: 4

Ingredients:

- 2 ripe bananas, mashed

- 2 eggs

- 1 cup gluten-free oat flour

- 1/2 cup unsweetened almond milk

- 1 tsp baking powder

- 1/4 tsp salt

- 1/2 tsp cinnamon

- 1/2 cup chopped walnuts

- 1 tablespoon maple syrup (for serving)

- Non-stick cooking spray

Preparation instructions:

1. In a large mixing bowl, combine the mashed bananas and eggs. Mix until well combined.

2. To the banana mixture, add the oat flour, almond milk, baking powder, salt, and cinnamon. Mix the batter until it's smooth.

3. Fold in the chopped walnuts.

4. Heat a non-stick skillet over medium heat and spray with non-stick cooking spray.

5. Pour 1/4 cup of batter onto the skillet for each pancake. Cook for 2-3 minutes on one side, or until bubbles form on the surface and the edges look set.

6. After flipping, cook the pancakes for a further two to three minutes, or until golden brown on the opposite side.

7. Serve hot with a drizzle of maple syrup.

Per serving: Calories: 280; Fat: 15g; Protein: 8g; Carbs: 32g; Sugar: 10g; Fiber: 4g

---

4. Quinoa Breakfast Bowl

Prep time: 10 minutes

Cook time: 20 minutes

Serves: 2

Ingredients:

- 1 cup quinoa, rinsed

- 2 cups water

- 1/4 teaspoon salt

- 1/2 tablespoon cinnamon

- 1 tablespoon maple syrup

- 1/4 cup almond milk

- 1/2 cup blueberries

- 1 banana, sliced

- 2 tablespoon chopped almonds

Directions:

1. In a medium saucepan, bring the 2 cups of water to a boil. Add the quinoa and salt, then reduce the heat to low. Cover and simmer for 15 minutes, or until the quinoa is tender and the water is absorbed.

2. Remove from heat and let it stand covered for 5 minutes. Fluff the quinoa with a fork.

3. Stir in the cinnamon, maple syrup, and almond milk, mixing well.

4. Divide the quinoa between two bowls. Top each bowl with blueberries, banana slices, and chopped almonds.

5. Serve warm, and enjoy your nutritious start to the day!

Per serving: Calories: 315; Fat: 7g; Protein: 9g; Carbs: 55g; Sugar: 15g; Fiber: 8g

---

5. Chia Seed Pudding with Berries

Prep time: 15 minutes

Cook time: 0 minutes (requires overnight refrigeration)

Serves: 2

Ingredients:

- 1/4 cup chia seeds

- 1 cup almond milk, unsweetened

- 1/2 teaspoon vanilla extract

- 1 tbsp maple syrup (optional, for sweetness)

- 1/2 cup mixed berries (strawberries, blueberries, raspberries), fresh or frozen

- A pinch of salt

Preparation instructions:

1. In a mixing bowl, combine the almond milk, vanilla extract, chia seeds, maple syrup (if using), and a pinch of salt. Stir well until the mixture is well combined.

2. Cover the bowl with a lid or plastic wrap and refrigerate overnight, or at least for 6 hours, allowing the chia seeds to swell and absorb the liquid, forming a pudding-like consistency.

3. Before serving, give the chia pudding a good stir to ensure it has thickened evenly. Adjust the sweetness if necessary by adding a little more maple syrup.

4. Serve the chia seed pudding in bowls or glasses and top with the mixed berries.

Per serving: Calories: 150; Fat: 7g; Protein: 4g; Carbs: 18g; Sugar: 8g (natural sugars from berries and optional maple syrup); Fiber: 9g

Difficulty rating: ★ ☆ ☆ ☆ ☆

Allergen information: Gluten-free, Dairy-free, Nut-free (ensure almond milk is produced in a nut-free facility if a nut allergy is a concern), Vegan

---

6. Sweet Potato Hash with Eggs

Prep time: 15 minutes

Cook time: 30 minutes

Serves: 4

Ingredients:

- 2 medium-sized sweet potatoes, chopped and skinned

- 1 tbsp garlic-infused olive oil

- 1 red bell pepper, diced

- 1 green bell pepper, diced

- 1/2 cup chopped green onions (green parts only)

- 1 teaspoon smoked paprika

- Salt and pepper, to taste

- 4 large eggs

- 2 tbsp fresh chives, chopped (garnish)

Preparation instructions:

1. Preheat the oven to 400°F (200°C).

2. On a baking sheet, toss the diced sweet potatoes with garlic-infused olive oil, smoked paprika, salt, and pepper. Spread in a single layer.

3. Roast in the preheated oven for 20 minutes, or until tender and golden, stirring halfway through.

4. While the sweet potatoes are roasting, heat a non-stick skillet over medium heat. Add a little olive oil and sauté the green onion, red bell pepper, and green bell pepper until softened, about 5-7 minutes.

5. Once the sweet potatoes are done, add them to the skillet with the sautéed vegetables, mixing well.

6. In the hash mixture, make four wells and crack one egg into each well. Place a lid on the skillet and cook on low heat for 5 to 8 minutes, or until the eggs set to your preference.

7. Garnish with chopped chives before serving.

Per serving: Calories: 250; Fat: 11g; Protein: 9g; Carbs: 30g; Sugar: 7g; Fiber: 5g

7. Greek Yogurt Parfait

Prep time: 10 minutes

Cook time: 0 minutes

Serves: 2

Ingredients:

- 1 cup lactose-free Greek yogurt

- 1/4 cup gluten-free granola

- 1/2 cup mixed berries (strawberries, blueberries, raspberries)

- 1 tablespoon maple syrup (optional)

- 1 teaspoon vanilla extract

- 1 tablespoon chia seeds (optional, extra fiber)

Preparation instructions:

1. In a small bowl, mix the lactose-free Greek yogurt with vanilla extract and maple syrup (if using) until well combined.

2. In serving glasses or bowls, layer half of the Greek yogurt mixture.

3. Add a layer of half the mixed berries over the yogurt.

4. Sprinkle half of the gluten-free granola over the berries.

5. With the remaining yogurt, granola, and berries, repeat the layering.

6. Top with chia seeds if desired for extra fiber.

7. Serve immediately or refrigerate until ready to serve.

Per serving: Calories: 220; Fat: 3g; Protein: 12g; Carbs: 36g; Sugar: 18g (natural sugars from berries and optional maple syrup); Fiber: 4g

Difficulty rating: ★☆☆☆☆

Allergen information: Gluten-free, Lactose-free. Please ensure all ingredients are suitable for your dietary needs.

---

8. Avocado and Egg Toast

Prep time: 10 minutes

Cook time: 5 minutes

Serves: 2

Ingredients:

- 1/4 ripe avocado (≈30g total, Low-FODMAP portion when divided)

- 2 slices of gluten-free bread

- 2 large eggs

- Salt and pepper, to taste

- 1 tablespoon olive oil

- Optional toppings: crushed red pepper flakes, fresh herbs (such as parsley or cilantro), sliced radishes

Preparation instructions:

1. Heat olive oil in a non-stick skillet over medium heat. Crack eggs into skillet and cook to your liking (2–3 minutes for sunny-side up). Season with salt and pepper.

2. Toast the gluten-free bread slices until golden and crisp.

3. Mash the avocado in a bowl, season with salt and pepper. Use only 1 tablespoon per toast to stay within Low-FODMAP limits.

4. Spread mashed avocado over each slice of toast.

5. Top with a cooked egg.

6. Add any optional toppings you like.

7. Serve immediately.

Per serving: ~270; Fat: 19g; Protein: 12g; Carbs: 17g; Sugar: 2g; Fiber: 5g

Difficulty rating: ★☆☆☆☆

---

9. Gluten-Free Waffles

Prep time: 10 minutes

Cook time: 15 minutes

Serves: 4

Ingredients:

- 1 cup gluten-free all-purpose flour

- 1 tablespoon granulated sugar

- 1 teaspoon baking powder

- 1/2 teaspoon baking soda

- 1/4 teaspoon salt

- 1 cup lactose-free milk

- 2 large eggs

- 2 tablespoons melted coconut oil, plus extra for greasing

- 1 teaspoon vanilla extract

Preparation instructions:

1. Mix the sugar, baking soda, baking powder, gluten-free flour, and salt in a sizable mixing bowl.

2. In another bowl, beat the eggs and then mix in the lactose-free milk, melted coconut oil, and vanilla extract.

3. Take care not to overmix while adding the wet and dry ingredients; whisk just until incorporated..

4. As directed by the manufacturer, preheat your waffle iron and give it a quick coat of coconut oil.

5. Pour enough batter onto the waffle iron to just cover the waffle grid.

6. Close the lid and cook until the waffle is golden and crisp, about 3-5 minutes.

7. Carefully remove the waffle and repeat with the remaining batter.

8. Serve warm with your choice of low-FODMAP toppings, such as maple syrup, fresh berries, or a dollop of lactose-free yogurt.

Per serving: Calories: 250; Fat: 11g; Protein: 6g; Carbs: 33g; Sugar: 6g; Fiber: 2g

Difficulty rating: ★★☆☆☆

---

10. Pumpkin Spice Smoothie

Prep time: 5 minutes

Cook time: 0 minutes

Serves: 2

Ingredients:

- 1 cup unsweetened almond milk

- 1/2 cup pumpkin puree (canned or fresh)

- 1 banana, frozen

- 1 tbsp maple syrup (optional)

- 1/2 teaspoon vanilla extract

- 3/4 teaspoon pumpkin pie spice

- 1/2 cup ice cubes

Preparation instructions:

1. In a blender, combine the almond milk, pumpkin puree, frozen banana, maple syrup (if using), vanilla extract, and pumpkin pie spice.

2. Blend on high until smooth and creamy.

3. Add the ice cubes and blend again until the smoothie reaches your desired consistency.

4. Pour into glasses and serve immediately.

Per serving: Calories: 145; Fat: 1.5g; Protein: 2g; Carbs: 31g; Sugar: 18g (0g added sugars, unless maple syrup is added); Fiber: 4g

---

11. Coconut Flour Muffins

Prep time: 15 minutes

Cook time: 20 minutes

Serves: 12 muffins

Ingredients:

- 1 cup coconut flour

- 1/2 teaspoon baking soda

- 1/4 teaspoon salt

- 6 large eggs

- 1/2 cup coconut oil, melted

- 1/2 cup maple syrup

- 1 teaspoon vanilla extract

- 1/2 cup unsweetened almond milk

- 1/2 cup blueberries (optional)

Preparation instructions:

1. Preheat your oven to 350°F (175°C) and line a muffin tin with paper liners or grease with coconut oil.

2. In a large bowl, whisk together the coconut flour, baking soda, and salt.

3. In a separate bowl, beat the eggs and then mix in the melted coconut oil, maple syrup, and vanilla extract until well combined.

4. Add the wet ingredients to the dry ingredients and stir until just combined. Gently fold in the almond milk until the batter is smooth. If using, fold in the blueberries.

5. Divide the batter evenly among the 12 muffin cups, filling each about two-thirds full.

6. A toothpick put into the center of a muffin should come out clean after 20 minutes of baking.

7. Let the muffins cool in the pan for 5 minutes, then transfer to a wire rack to cool completely.

Per serving: Calories: 190; Fat: 14g; Protein: 5g; Carbs: 12g; Sugar: 7g; Fiber: 5g

Difficulty rating: ★★★☆☆

12. Scrambled Tofu with Vegetables

Prep time: 10 minutes

Cook time: 15 minutes

Serves: 2

Ingredients:

- 14 oz firm tofu, drained and crumbled

- 1 tablespoon olive oil

- 1/2 cup red bell pepper, diced

- 1/2 cup zucchini, diced

- 1/4 cup carrots, diced

- 1/4 cup spinach, chopped

- 1/4 teaspoon turmeric (for color)

- Salt and pepper, to taste

- 1 tbs nutritional yeast (optional, cheesy taste)

- 1/4 cup lactose-free milk or almond milk

- Fresh herbs (such as parsley or chives), for garnish

Directions:

1. Heat olive oil in a large skillet over medium heat.

2. Add the red bell pepper, zucchini, and carrots to the skillet. Sauté for 5-7 minutes, or until vegetables are tender.

3. Stir in the crumbled tofu and turmeric, mixing well to combine. Cook for another 5 minutes, stirring occasionally.

4. Season with salt and pepper. If using, sprinkle nutritional yeast over the mixture and stir in the lactose-free milk or almond milk to add moisture and a creamy texture.

5. Finally, add the chopped spinach and cook for an additional 2-3 minutes, or until the spinach has wilted.

6. Serve hot, garnished with fresh herbs.

Per serving: Calories: 220; Fat: 13g; Protein: 18g; Carbs: 9g; Sugar: 3g; Fiber: 4g

Difficulty rating: ★☆☆☆☆

13. Buckwheat Porridge

Prep time: 5 minutes

Cook time: 15 minutes

Serves: 2

Ingredients:

- 1 cup buckwheat groats

- 2 cups water or low-FODMAP milk alternative (e.g., almond milk)

- 1/4 teaspoon salt

- 1 tablespoon maple syrup (optional)

- 1/2 teaspoon cinnamon

- Fresh berries (for topping)

- Sliced bananas (for topping)

- A handful of walnuts (for topping)

Preparation instructions:

1. Rinse the buckwheat groats under cold water until the water runs clear.

2. In a medium saucepan, bring the water or low-FODMAP milk alternative to a boil.

3. Add the buckwheat groats and salt to the boiling water or milk, then reduce the heat to low.

4. Cover and simmer for 10-15 minutes, or until the groats are tender and the liquid is mostly absorbed.

5. Remove from heat and let it stand covered for 5 minutes.

6. Stir in the maple syrup and cinnamon.

7. Serve hot, topped with fresh berries, sliced bananas, and a handful of walnuts.

Nutritional values per serving: Calories: 350; Fat: 5g; Protein: 12g; Carbs: 68g; Sugar: 9g (0g if maple syrup is not added); Fiber: 10g

Difficulty rating: ★☆☆☆☆

Allergen information: Gluten-free, Dairy-free, Soy-free. Please ensure the milk alternative and toppings used are suitable for your specific dietary needs.

---

14. Blueberry Cinnamon Breakfast Bars

Prep time: 15 minutes

Cook time: 30 minutes

Serves: 12

Ingredients:

- 2 cups gluten-free rolled oats

- 1 tsp baking powder

- 1 ½ tsp ground cinnamon

- ¼ tsp salt

- 1 cup unsweetened almond milk

- ¼ cup maple syrup

- 1 large egg

- 2 tbsp melted coconut oil

- 1 tsp vanilla extract

- 1 cup blueberries

- ½ cup chopped walnuts (optional)

Preparation instructions:

1. Preheat your oven to 350°F (175°C). Line an 8-inch square baking dish with parchment paper.

2. In a large bowl, mix together the oats, baking powder, cinnamon, and salt.

3. In another bowl, whisk together the almond milk, maple syrup, egg, melted coconut oil, and vanilla extract.

4. Pour the wet ingredients into the dry ingredients and stir until combined.

5. Fold in the blueberries and walnuts, if using.

6. Spread the mixture evenly into the prepared baking dish.

7. Bake for 30 minutes, or until the top is golden and a toothpick inserted into the center comes out clean.

8. Let the bars cool in the pan for 10 minutes, then transfer to a wire rack to cool completely before cutting into bars.

Per serving: Calories: 150; Fat: 7g; Protein: 4g; Carbs: 20g; Sugar: 7g; Fiber: 3g

Difficulty rating: ★☆☆☆☆

---

15. Smoked Salmon and Cream Cheese Bagel

Prep time: 10 minutes

Cook time: 0 minutes

Serves: 2

Ingredients:

- 2 gluten-free bagels, halved

- 4 oz smoked salmon

- 2 tbsp cream cheese, lactose-free

- 1/2 cup chopped green onions (green parts only)

- 1 tbsp capers, drained

- 2 slices of tomato

- Fresh dill, for garnish

- Freshly ground black pepper, to taste

Preparation instructions:

1. Toast the gluten-free bagels to your desired level of crispiness.

2. Spread 1 tablespoon of lactose-free cream cheese on each bagel half.

3. Place an equal amount of smoked salmon on top of the cream cheese on each bagel half.

4. Add a few slices of green onions and a slice of tomato to each bagel half.

5. Sprinkle capers over the top.

6. Garnish with fresh dill and a sprinkle of freshly ground black pepper.

7. Serve immediately and enjoy.

Per serving: Calories: 320; Fat: 9g; Protein: 22g; Carbs: 41g; Sugar: 6g; Fiber: 3g

Light Meals & Snacks

16. Chicken and Veggie Lettuce Boats

Prep time: 20 minutes

Cook time: 10 minutes

Serves: 4

Ingredients:

- 1 lb chicken breast, thinly sliced

- 1 tbsp garlic-infused olive oil

- 1 tbsp soy sauce (gluten-free, low-sodium)

- 1 teaspoon ginger, grated

- 1/4 teaspoon chili flakes (optional)

- Salt and pepper, to taste

- 8 large lettuce leaves (e.g., Bibb or iceberg)

- 1 carrot, julienned

- 1/4 cucumber, julienned

- 1/4 red bell pepper, julienned

- 2 tbsp fresh cilantro, chopped

- 2 tbsp green onions, green parts only, sliced

Preparation instructions:

1. In a large bowl, combine the chicken slices with garlic-infused olive oil, soy sauce, grated ginger, chili flakes (if using), salt, and pepper. Mix well to ensure the chicken is evenly coated.

2. Heat a non-stick skillet over medium-high heat. Add the chicken mixture to the skillet and cook for about 5-7 minutes, or until the chicken is fully cooked and slightly browned. Remove from heat.

3. Prepare the lettuce leaves by rinsing and drying them thoroughly.

4. To assemble the wraps, divide the cooked chicken evenly among the lettuce leaves.

5. Top the chicken with julienned carrot, cucumber, red bell pepper, chopped cilantro, and sliced green onions.

6. Serve immediately, allowing diners to fold their lettuce wraps as they eat.

Per serving: Calories: 165; Fat: 4g; Protein: 26g; Carbs: 5g; Sugar: 2g; Fiber: 1g

Prep time: 15 minutes

Cook time: 10 minutes

Serves: 4

Ingredients:

- 2 medium zucchinis, grated

- 1/4 cup almond flour

- 2 large eggs, beaten

- 1/4 cup grated Parmesan cheese (hard, aged)

- 1 tbsp fresh chives, chopped

- Salt and pepper, to taste

- 2 tbsp garlic-infused olive oil, for frying

Preparation instructions:

1. Place the grated zucchini in a colander, sprinkle with salt, and let it sit for 10 minutes to draw out moisture. Squeeze the excess water from the zucchini using a clean kitchen towel.

2. In a large bowl, combine the drained zucchini, almond flour, beaten eggs, Parmesan cheese, chives, and season with salt and pepper. Mix until well combined.

3. Heat the garlic-infused olive oil in a large skillet over medium heat.

4. Using a spatula, flatten 1/4 cup of the zucchini mixture into a fritter in the skillet. Cook until crispy and golden brown, 3 to 5 minutes per side.

5. Transfer the fritters to a plate lined with paper towels to drain any excess oil.

6. Serve warm.

Per serving: Calories: 180; Fat: 14g; Protein: 8g; Carbs: 6g; Sugar: 2g; Fiber: 2g

Difficulty rating: ★★☆☆☆

Prep time: 15 minutes

Cook time: 0 minutes

Serves: 4

Ingredients:

- 2 large cucumbers, thinly sliced

- 1/4 cup fresh dill, chopped

- 2 tbsp olive oil

- 2 tbsp white wine vinegar

- 1 tbsp lemon juice

- 1/2 teaspoon salt

- 1/4 teaspoon black pepper

- 1 tbsp Dijon mustard

- 1 tbsp maple syrup (optional, for sweetness)

Preparation instructions:

1. In a large mixing bowl, combine the thinly sliced cucumbers and chopped fresh dill.

2. In a small bowl, whisk together olive oil, white wine vinegar, lemon juice, salt, black pepper, Dijon mustard, and maple syrup (if using) until well blended.

3. Pour the dressing over the cucumber and dill mixture. Toss gently to ensure all the cucumber slices are evenly coated with the dressing.

4. Cover and refrigerate for at least 1 hour before serving, allowing the flavors to meld together.

5. Toss again gently before serving. Adjust seasoning if necessary.

Per serving: Calories: 80; Fat: 7g; Protein: 1g; Carbohydrates: 4g; Sugar: 2g; Fiber: 1g

19. Turkey and Cream Cheese Roll-Ups

Difficulty rating: ★☆☆☆☆

Prep time: 15 minutes

Cook time: 0 minutes

Serves: 4

Ingredients:

- 8 slices of turkey breast, thinly sliced

- 1/2 cup lactose-free cream cheese

- 1 tablespoon lime juice

- 1/4 teaspoon salt

- 1/4 teaspoon black pepper

- 1/2 cup baby spinach leaves

- 1/4 cup shredded carrots

- 1/4 cup cucumber, thinly sliced

- 1/4 cup red bell pepper, thinly sliced

Preparation instructions:

1. In a small bowl, mix the lactose-free cream cheese with lime juice, salt, and pepper until smooth.

2. Lay out the turkey breast slices on a flat surface.

3. Spread the cream cheese mixture evenly over each turkey slice.

4. Place a few spinach leaves, shredded carrots, cucumber slices, and red bell pepper strips on one end of each turkey slice.

5. Carefully roll up the turkey slices tightly, starting from the end with the vegetables.

6. Secure each roll-up with a toothpick if necessary.

7. Serve immediately or chill in the refrigerator until ready to serve.

Per serving: Calories: 210; Fat: 13g; Protein: 20g; Carbs: 9g; Sugar: 2g; Fiber: 6g

20. Carrot and Ginger Soup

Prep time: 15 minutes

Cook time: 25 minutes

Serves: 4

Ingredients:

- 1 tablespoon garlic-infused olive oil

- 1 pound carrots, peeled and diced

- 2 tablespoons ginger, finely grated

- 4 cups low-FODMAP vegetable broth

- 1 teaspoon turmeric

- Salt and pepper, to taste

- 1/4 cup lactose-free cream (optional, garnish)

- Fresh herbs (parsley or chives), for garnish

Preparation instructions:

1. The garlic-infused olive oil should be heated over medium heat in a big pot.

2. Add the diced carrots and grated ginger to the pot, sautéing for 5 minutes until the carrots start to soften.

3. Pour in the low-FODMAP vegetable broth and add the turmeric. Stir well to combine.

4. Bring the mixture to a boil, then reduce the heat and simmer for 20 minutes, or until the carrots are very tender.

5. Puree the soup with an immersion blender until it's smooth. As an alternative, move the soup to a blender and process the soup in portions. When combining hot liquids, exercise caution.

6. Season the soup with salt and pepper to taste.

7. Serve hot, garnished with a drizzle of lactose-free cream and fresh herbs if desired.

Per serving: Calories: 120; Fat: 5g; Protein: 2g; Carbs: 18g; Sugar: 8g; Fiber: 4g

Difficulty rating: ★☆☆☆☆

---

21. Zucchini and Turkey Roll-Ups

Prep time: 20 minutes

Cook time: 10 minutes

Serves: 4

Ingredients:

- 2 large zucchinis, thinly sliced lengthwise

- 1 tablespoon garlic-infused olive oil

- 1 pound ground turkey

- 1 teaspoon dried oregano

- 1 teaspoon dried basil

- 1/2 teaspoon salt

- 1/4 teaspoon ground black pepper

- 1/2 cup diced tomatoes (ensure no onion or garlic for low-FODMAP)

- 1/2 cup lactose-free shredded mozzarella

- 1/4 cup chopped fresh parsley

Preparation instructions:

1. Preheat your grill to medium-high heat.

2. Brush the zucchini slices with garlic-infused olive oil and grill for 2-3 minutes on each side, until tender and grill marks appear. Set aside to cool slightly.

3. In a large skillet, heat the remaining garlic-infused olive oil over medium heat. Add the ground turkey, oregano, basil, salt, and pepper.

Break up the turkey with a spoon while it cooks and continue to cook until it is browned and cooked through.

4. Stir in the diced tomatoes and cook for another 2-3 minutes.

5. At one end of each zucchini slice, place a dollop of the turkey mixture, then tightly roll each slice. Secure with toothpicks if necessary.

6. Arrange the roll-ups on a serving platter and top with shredded mozzarella cheese and chopped fresh parsley.

7. Serve warm or at room temperature.

Per serving: Calories: 280; Fat: 15g; Protein: 25g; Carbs: 10g; Sugar: 4g; Fiber: 2g

Difficulty rating: ★★☆☆☆

22. Mexican Quinoa Salad

Prep time: 20 minutes

Cook time: 15 minutes

Serves: 4

Ingredients:

- 1 cup quinoa

- 2 cups water

- 3/4 cup canned lentils, rinsed and drained

- 1 red bell pepper, diced

- 1/4 cup fresh cilantro, chopped

- 1/4 cup lime juice

- 2 tablespoons olive oil

- 1/2 teaspoon ground cumin

- Salt and pepper, to taste

- Optional: 2 tablespoons avocado (≈30g), diced – Low-FODMAP portion for 4 servings

- 1/4 cup green onions, sliced (green parts only)

Preparation instructions:

1. Boil two cups of water in a medium pot. Add the quinoa, cover, lower the heat to a simmer, and cook until the water is completely absorbed, about 15 minutes. Take off the heat, cover for five minutes, fluff with a fork, and allow to cool.

2. In a large mixing bowl, combine the cooled quinoa with canned lentils, diced red bell pepper, and chopped cilantro.

3. In a separate small bowl, whisk together lime juice, olive oil, ground cumin, salt, and pepper to make the dressing.

4. Pour the dressing over the quinoa mixture, stirring gently to ensure everything is evenly coated.

5. Carefully fold in the diced avocado and sliced green onions.

6. Serve chilled or at room temperature.

Per serving: Calories: 290; Fat: 12g; Protein: 9g; Carbs: 35g; Fiber: 8g

---

23. Baked Sweet Potato Fries

Prep time: 10 minutes

Cook time: 25 minutes

Serves: 4

Ingredients:

- 2 large sweet potatoes, peeled and cut into 1/4-inch thick fries

- 2 tablespoons garlic-infused olive oil

- 1/2 teaspoon paprika

- Salt and pepper, to taste

Preparation instructions:

1. Preheat the oven to 425°F (220°C). Line a baking sheet with parchment paper.

2. Combine the sweet potato fries, paprika, garlic-infused olive oil, salt, and pepper in a big bowl and toss until well coated.

3. To ensure even cooking, arrange the fries on the prepared baking sheet in a single layer, being careful not to touch.

4. Bake in the preheated oven for 25 minutes, or until crispy and golden brown, turning the fries halfway through the cooking time.

5. Remove from the oven and let cool slightly before serving.

Per serving: Calories: 200; Fat: 7g; Protein: 2g; Carbs: 34g; Sugar: 7g; Fiber: 5g

Difficulty rating: ★☆☆☆☆

24. Zucchini Hummus and Veggie Platter

Prep time: 20 minutes

Cook time: 0 minutes

Serves: 4

Ingredients:

- 2 medium zucchinis, peeled and chopped
- 2 tablespoons tahini
- 2 tablespoons lemon juice
- 1/4 teaspoon salt
- 2 tablespoons garlic-infused olive oil
- 1/4 teaspoon paprika (optional, for garnish)
- 1 cucumber, sliced into rounds
- 2 carrots, peeled and cut into sticks
- 1 bell pepper (red or yellow), sliced
- 10 cherry tomatoes, halved
- 1/4 cup olives, pitted

Preparation instructions:

1. In a food processor, combine the chopped zucchini, tahini, lemon juice, and salt. Blend until smooth.

2. While blending, slowly add the garlic-infused olive oil until the mixture is creamy.

3. Transfer the hummus to a serving bowl. If desired, sprinkle paprika on top for garnish.

4. Arrange the cucumber rounds, carrot sticks, bell pepper slices, cherry tomatoes, and olives on a large platter around the bowl of hummus.

5. Serve immediately, allowing guests to dip the veggies into the hummus.

Per serving: Calories: 170; Fat: 12g; Protein: 3g; Carbs: 12g; Sugar: 3g; Fiber: 4g

25. Shrimp with Pineapple Salsa

Prep time: 20 minutes

Cook time: 0 minutes

Serves: 4

Ingredients:

- 1 lb cooked shrimp, tails removed and chopped
- 1 cup fresh pineapple, diced
- 1/2 red bell pepper, finely diced
- 1/2 cup green onions (green parts only), finely chopped
- 1/4 cup fresh cilantro, chopped
- Juice of 1 lime
- Salt and pepper, to taste
- Optional: 2 tablespoons avocado (≈30g total), diced
- Tortilla chips, for serving (ensure gluten-free for a fully low-FODMAP meal)

Preparation instructions:

1. In a large bowl, combine shrimp, diced pineapple, red bell pepper, green onion tops, and cilantro.

2. Add lime juice, season with salt and pepper, and gently toss to combine.

3. If using avocado, fold it in just before serving.

4. Serve chilled with gluten-free tortilla chips.

Per serving: Calories: 210; Fat: 4g; Protein: 24g; Carbs: 17g; Sugar: 8g; Fiber: 2g

Difficulty rating: ★☆☆☆☆

26. Cottage Cheese and Pineapple Bowl

Prep time: 5 minutes

Cook time: 0 minutes

Serves: 1

Ingredients:

- 1/2 cup lactose-free cottage cheese

- 1/2 cup pineapple chunks, fresh or canned in their own juice

- 1 tablespoon shredded coconut, unsweetened

- 1 teaspoon chia seeds

- 1 tablespoon sliced almonds

Preparation instructions:

1. Place the lactose-free cottage cheese at the bottom of a serving bowl.

2. Top the cottage cheese with pineapple chunks.

3. Sprinkle shredded coconut, chia seeds, and sliced almonds over the pineapple.

4. Serve immediately or chill in the refrigerator for 30 minutes before serving for a refreshing snack.

Per serving: Calories: 200; Fat: 8g; Protein: 14g; Carbs: 18g; Sugar: 12g; Fiber: 3g

---

27. Rice Paper Veggie Rolls

Prep time: 20 minutes

Cook time: 0 minutes

Serves: 4

Ingredients:

- 8 rice paper wrappers

- 1 cup lettuce, shredded

- 1 carrot, julienned

- 1 cucumber, julienned

- 1/4 red bell pepper, julienned

- 1/4 yellow bell pepper, julienned

- 1/2 cup purple cabbage, thinly sliced

- 1/4 cup fresh cilantro leaves

- 1/4 cup fresh mint leaves

- 1/4 cup cooked rice vermicelli noodles (optional)

- Warm water for softening rice paper

Preparation instructions:

1. Tip in a big dish of warm water. To make one rice paper wrapper just soft, dip it into the water for ten to fifteen seconds. Spread out the wrapper using a fresh, somewhat moist cloth.

2. In the center of the wrapper, place a small amount of lettuce, carrots, cucumber, red and yellow bell peppers, purple cabbage, cilantro, mint, and rice vermicelli noodles (if using).

3. The rice paper wrapper should be folded with the bottom half covering the filling. Fold the sides of the wrapper in, making sure to hold everything firmly in place. To create a tight roll, roll the wrapper upwards next. Continue adding ingredients and wrappings.

4. Serve immediately with your choice of low-FODMAP dipping sauce.

Per serving: Calories: 100; Fat: 0g; Protein: 2g; Carbs: 22g; Sugar: 2g; Fiber: 2g

Difficulty rating: ★☆☆☆☆

Lunches

28. Grilled Chicken Caesar Salad

Prep time: 20 minutes

Cook time: 10 minutes

Serves: 4

Ingredients:

- 4 boneless, skinless chicken breasts
- 1 tablespoon garlic-infused olive oil
- Salt and pepper, to taste
- 8 cups romaine lettuce, chopped
- 1/2 cup cherry tomatoes, halved
- 1/4 cup shaved Parmesan cheese
- 1/4 cup low-FODMAP Caesar dressing
- 1 tablespoon lemon juice
- 1/2 cup gluten-free croutons

Preparation instructions:

1. Preheat the grill to medium-high heat.

2. Brush the chicken breasts with garlic-infused olive oil and season with salt and pepper.

3. Grill the chicken for 5 minutes on each side, or until fully cooked through. Remove from the grill and let it rest for a few minutes before slicing thinly.

4. In a large bowl, combine the chopped romaine lettuce, cherry tomatoes, and shaved Parmesan cheese.

5. Add the sliced chicken to the salad.

6. In a small bowl, whisk together the low-FODMAP Caesar dressing and lemon juice. Drizzle over the salad and toss to combine.

7. Top the salad with gluten-free croutons before serving.

Per serving: Calories: 320; Fat: 14g; Protein: 36g; Carbs: 12g; Sugar: 3g; Fiber: 3g

---

29. Turkey and Swiss Sandwich

Prep time: 10 minutes

Cook time: 0 minutes

Serves: 2

Ingredients:

- 4 slices gluten-free bread
- 4 slices deli turkey breast (no garlic or onion)
- 2 slices Swiss cheese
- 1/4 cup baby spinach leaves
- 1/4 cup grated carrot
- 2 tbsp mustard (ensure low-FODMAP)
- 2 tbsp mayonnaise (ensure low-FODMAP)
- Butter or olive oil for toasting bread (optional)

Preparation instructions:

1. If desired, lightly butter or brush olive oil on one side of each bread slice and toast in a skillet over medium heat until golden brown. Set aside.

2. Spread mustard on the non-toasted side of two bread slices.

3. Spread mayonnaise on the non-toasted side of the remaining two bread slices.

4. On top of the mustard-spread slices, layer each with 2 slices of turkey and 1 slice of Swiss cheese.

5. Add a layer of baby spinach leaves and grated carrot over the Swiss cheese.

6. Top each sandwich with the mayonnaise-spread bread slices, toasted side out, if applicable.

7. Cut sandwiches in half and serve immediately.

Per serving: Calories: 380; Fat: 20g; Protein: 25g; Carbs: 28g; Sugar: 4g; Fiber: 3g

---

30. Quinoa and Roasted Vegetable Bowl

Prep time: 20 minutes

Cook time: 25 minutes

Serves: 4

Ingredients:

- 1 cup quinoa

- 2 cups water

- 1 small zucchini, diced

- 1 red bell pepper, diced

- 1 yellow bell pepper, diced

- 1 medium carrot, peeled and diced

- 1 tablespoon olive oil

- 1 teaspoon dried oregano

- 1/2 teaspoon salt

- 1/4 teaspoon black pepper

- 1 tablespoon balsamic vinegar

- 1/4 cup fresh parsley, chopped

Preparation instructions:

1. Preheat the oven to 400°F (200°C). Line a baking sheet with parchment paper.

2. Heat the two cups of water in a medium-sized saucepan until it boils. Once all of the water has been absorbed, add the quinoa, lower the heat to low, cover, and simmer for 15 minutes. After removing from the fire and standing for five minutes, fluff with a fork.

3. While the quinoa is cooking, toss the zucchini, red and yellow bell peppers, and carrot with olive oil, oregano, salt, and pepper on the prepared baking sheet. Spread the vegetables in an even layer.

4. Roast the vegetables in the preheated oven for 20 minutes, stirring halfway through, or until they are soft and beginning to caramelize.

5. In a large bowl, combine the cooked quinoa and roasted vegetables. Drizzle with balsamic vinegar and add the fresh parsley. Toss everything together until well mixed.

6. Serve warm or at room temperature.

Per serving: Calories: 220; Fat: 7g; Protein: 6g; Carbs: 35g; Sugar: 5g; Fiber: 5g

Difficulty rating: ★★☆☆☆

---

31. Chicken Herb Salad with Lemon Vinaigrette

Prep time: 20 minutes

Cook time: 10 minutes

Serves: 4

Ingredients:

- 2 large chicken breasts, grilled and sliced

- 4 cups mixed greens (such as spinach and arugula)

- 1/2 cucumber, thinly sliced

- 1/2 cup chopped green onions (green parts only)

- 1/4 cup cherry tomatoes, halved

- 2 tablespoons olive oil

- 1 tablespoon balsamic vinegar

- Salt and pepper, to taste

- 1 tablespoon fresh lemon juice

- 1/4 cup fresh cilantro, chopped

Preparation instructions:

1. Grill the chicken breasts over medium heat until fully cooked, about 5 minutes per side. Let them cool slightly before slicing.

2. In a large salad bowl, combine the mixed greens, cucumber, cherry tomatoes, and green onion tops.

3. In a small bowl, whisk together olive oil, balsamic vinegar, lemon juice, salt, and pepper to create the dressing.

4. Add the sliced grilled chicken to the salad bowl.

5. Pour the dressing over the salad and toss gently to combine everything well.

6. Garnish with fresh cilantro before serving.

Per serving: Calories: 240; Fat: 12g; Protein: 26g; Carbs: 6g; Sugar: 3g; Fiber: 2g

32. Lentil and Spinach Soup

Prep time: 10 minutes

Cook time: 25 minutes

Serves: 4

Ingredients:

- 1 tablespoon garlic-infused olive oil

- 2 cups water

- 1 cup low-FODMAP vegetable broth

- 1 cup dried red lentils, rinsed

- 2 cups spinach, roughly chopped

- 1 carrot, peeled and diced

- 1 teaspoon ground cumin

- 1 teaspoon ground coriander

- 1/2 teaspoon turmeric

- 1/4 teaspoon smoked paprika

- Salt and pepper, to taste

- 1 tablespoon lemon juice

- 2 tablespoons fresh cilantro, chopped (for garnish)

Preparation instructions:

1. Heat the garlic-infused olive oil in a large pot over medium heat.

2. Add the diced carrot to the pot and sauté for 2-3 minutes until slightly softened.

3. Add the smoked paprika, turmeric, ground coriander, and cumin. Simmer for one minute, or until aromatic.

4. Pour in the water and low-FODMAP vegetable broth, then add the rinsed red lentils. Bring to a boil.

5. Lentils should be tender after 20 minutes of simmering, covered, with reduced heat.

6. Add the chopped spinach to the pot and cook for an additional 2-3 minutes, until the spinach has wilted.

7. Remove from heat and stir in the lemon juice. Season with salt and pepper to taste.

8. Serve hot, garnished with fresh cilantro.

Per serving: Calories: 220; Fat: 4g; Protein: 14g; Carbs: 33g; Sugar: 3g; Fiber: 16g

Difficulty rating: ★☆☆☆☆

---

33. Tuna Salad Lettuce Wraps

Prep time: 15 minutes

Cook time: 0 minutes

Serves: 4

Ingredients:

- 2 cans (5 ounces each) tuna in water, drained

- 1/4 cup mayonnaise (low-FODMAP alternative)

- 1 tablespoon Dijon mustard

- 1/4 cup diced cucumber

- 1/4 cup diced red bell pepper

- 1 tablespoon chopped fresh chives

- 1 tablespoon chopped fresh dill

- Salt and pepper, to taste

- 8 large lettuce leaves (e.g., Bibb or Romaine)

Preparation instructions:

1. In a medium bowl, mix together the drained tuna, mayonnaise, Dijon mustard, diced cucumber, diced red bell pepper, chopped chives, and dill. Season with salt and pepper to taste.

2. Carefully wash the lettuce leaves and pat them dry with paper towels.

3. Place a portion of the tuna salad onto the center of each lettuce leaf.

4. Fold the lettuce around the filling to create a wrap. Serve immediately.

Nutritional values per serving: Calories: 180; Fat: 10g; Protein: 20g; Carbs: 4g; Sugar: 2g; Fiber: 1g

34. Vegetable and Hummus Wrap

Prep time: 15 minutes

Cook time: 0 minutes

Serves: 2

Ingredients:

- 2 gluten-free tortillas

- 1/2 cup homemade or store-bought low-FODMAP hummus

- 1 cup mixed greens (such as spinach and arugula)

- 1/2 cucumber, thinly sliced

- 1/2 red bell pepper, julienned

- 1/4 cup shredded carrots

- 1/4 cup alfalfa sprouts

- 2 tablespoons pumpkin seeds

- Salt and pepper, to taste

Preparation instructions:

1. Lay out the gluten-free tortillas on a clean, flat surface.

2. Each tortilla should have a quarter cup of hummus evenly spread over it, with a tiny border remaining around the borders.

3. On one half of each tortilla, layer the mixed greens, cucumber slices, julienned red bell pepper, shredded carrots, and alfalfa sprouts.

4. Sprinkle pumpkin seeds over the vegetables, and season with salt and pepper to taste.

5. Carefully fold the tortillas in half over the fillings, then roll tightly from one end to the other, ensuring the wrap is secure but not so tight that it tears.

6. Cut each wrap in half diagonally and serve immediately, or wrap tightly in foil to take on the go.

Per serving: Calories: 320; Fat: 15g; Protein: 12g; Carbs: 40g; Sugar: 5g; Fiber: 8g

Difficulty rating: ★☆☆☆☆

---

35. Chicken and Rice Soup

Prep time: 15 minutes

Cook time: 35 minutes

Serves: 4

Ingredients:

- 1 tablespoon garlic-infused olive oil

- 2 chicken breasts, diced

- 6 cups low-FODMAP chicken broth

- 1 cup cooked white rice

- 1 cup carrots, peeled and sliced

- 1/2 cup sliced green onions (green parts only)

- 1 teaspoon dried thyme

- 1 teaspoon dried parsley

- Salt and pepper, to taste

Preparation instructions:

1. In a large pot, warm the garlic-infused oil over medium heat. Add the chopped chicken breasts and heat for 5 to 7 minutes, or until browned all over.

2. Pour the low-FODMAP chicken broth into the pot and bring to a boil.

3. Add the cooked white rice, sliced carrots, chopped green onions, dried thyme, and dried

parsley to the pot. Reduce the heat to low, cover, and simmer for 25 minutes, or until the carrots are tender.

4. Season the soup with salt and pepper to taste.

5. Serve hot, garnished with additional green onion tops if desired.

Per serving: Calories: 250; Fat: 5g; Protein: 22g; Carbs: 30g; Sugar: 3g; Fiber: 2g

Difficulty rating: ★ ☆ ☆ ☆ ☆

---

36. Mediterranean Veggie Salad

Prep time: 15 minutes

Cook time: 0 minutes

Serves: 4

Ingredients:

- 1 cup cherry tomatoes, halved

- 1 cucumber, diced

- ½ cup red bell pepper, diced

- ½ cup zucchini, diced

- 1/2 cup green onions (green tops only), finely chopped

- 1/4 cup Kalamata olives, pitted and halved

- 1/4 cup crumbled feta cheese (lactose-free if needed)

- 2 tablespoons fresh parsley, chopped

- 2 tablespoons fresh mint, chopped

- 3 tablespoons extra virgin olive oil

- 1 tablespoon lemon juice

- 1/2 teaspoon dried oregano

- Salt and pepper, to taste

Preparation instructions:

1. In a large mixing bowl, combine the cherry tomatoes, cucumber, red bell pepper, zucchini, green onions, olives, feta, parsley, and mint.

2. In a small bowl, whisk together the olive oil, lemon juice, oregano, salt, and pepper.

3. Drizzle over the salad and toss gently to combine.

4. Let sit for 10 minutes before serving to blend the flavors.

Per serving: ~190; Fat: 14g; Protein: 4g; Carbs: 9g; Sugar: 4g; Fiber: 2g

Allergen Info: Gluten-free, Nut-free, Dairy-free option (omit feta or use dairy-free cheese)

---

37. Beef and Broccoli Delight

Prep time: 15 minutes

Cook time: 10 minutes

Serves: 4

Ingredients:

- 1 lb beef sirloin, thinly sliced

- 2 cups broccoli florets

- 1 tablespoon garlic-infused olive oil

- 2 tablespoons low-sodium soy sauce (ensure gluten-free if necessary)

- 1 tablespoon sesame oil

- 1 tablespoon ginger, grated

- 1/4 cup water

- 1 tablespoon cornstarch

- 1/4 teaspoon red pepper flakes (optional)

- Salt and pepper, to taste

- 1 tablespoon green onions, green parts only, sliced (for garnish)

- 1 teaspoon sesame seeds (for garnish)

Preparation instructions:

1. In a small bowl, whisk together the soy sauce, sesame oil, ginger, water, cornstarch, and red pepper flakes (if using) to create the sauce. Set aside.

2. Heat the garlic-infused olive oil in a large skillet or wok over medium-high heat.

3. Add the beef slices to the skillet and cook for 2-3 minutes, or until they start to brown. Take out of the skillet and place the beef aside.

4. In the same skillet, add the broccoli florets and stir-fry for about 4 minutes, or until they are tender but still crisp.

5. Put the steak back in the skillet. After thoroughly combining the sauce with the beef and broccoli, pour it over them. Simmer for an additional two minutes, or until the beef is cooked through and the sauce has thickened.

6. Season with salt and pepper to taste.

7. Garnish with sliced green onions and sesame seeds before serving.

Per serving: Calories: 250; Fat: 14g; Protein: 26g; Carbs: 8g; Sugar: 2g; Fiber: 2g

Difficulty rating: ★★☆☆☆

38. Shrimp and Quinoa Salad

Prep time: 20 minutes

Cook time: 15 minutes

Serves: 4

Ingredients:

- 1 cup quinoa

- 2 cups water

- 1 lb shrimp, peeled and deveined

- 1 tablespoon garlic-infused olive oil

- 1 red bell pepper, diced

- 1 cucumber, diced

- 1/4 cup fresh parsley, chopped

- 1/4 cup fresh mint, chopped

- Juice of 1 lemon

- Salt and pepper, to taste

Preparation instructions:

1. Rinse quinoa under cold water until the water runs clear. In a medium saucepan, bring 2 cups of

water to a boil. Add quinoa, reduce heat to low, cover, and simmer for 15 minutes or until all water is absorbed. Remove from heat and let it stand for 5 minutes, then fluff with a fork.

2. As the quinoa cooks, place a large skillet over medium heat with the garlic-infused olive oil. When the shrimp turn pink and opaque, add them and fry for two to three minutes on each side. To taste, add salt and pepper for seasoning. Take off the heat.

3. In a large bowl, combine cooked quinoa, cooked shrimp, red bell pepper, cucumber, parsley, mint, and lemon juice. Toss everything together until well mixed. Season with salt and pepper to taste.

4. Serve the salad either chilled or at room temperature.

Per serving: Calories: 290; Fat: 8g; Protein: 28g; Carbs: 27g; Sugar: 3g; Fiber: 4g

---

Prep time: 15 minutes

Cook time: 10 minutes

Serves: 2

Ingredients:

- 4 large eggs

- 2 tablespoons lactose-free mayonnaise

- 1 teaspoon Dijon mustard

- 1/4 teaspoon paprika

- Salt and pepper, to taste

- 4 slices gluten-free bread, toasted

- Lettuce leaves

- Sliced tomato

Preparation instructions:

1. Put the eggs in a pot and pour cold water over them. Over high heat, bring to a boil, cover, turn off the heat, and let stand for eight to ten minutes. Once drained, chill in ice water. Chop and peel the eggs.

2. In a bowl, mix the chopped eggs with lactose-free mayonnaise, Dijon mustard, paprika, salt, and pepper.

3. Divide the egg mixture evenly among two slices of toasted gluten-free bread.

4. Add lettuce leaves and sliced tomato on top of the egg mixture.

5. Cover with the remaining slices of toast.

6. Cut each sandwich in half and serve immediately.

Per serving: Calories: 350; Fat: 20g; Protein: 19g; Carbs: 25g; Sugar: 4g; Fiber: 3g

40. Roasted Vegetable and Goat Cheese Salad

Prep time: 20 minutes

Cook time: 25 minutes

Serves: 4

Ingredients:

- 2 medium zucchinis, sliced

- 1 red bell pepper, sliced

- 1 yellow bell pepper, sliced

- 1 medium eggplant, sliced

- 2 tablespoons olive oil

- Salt and pepper, to taste

- 4 ounces goat cheese, crumbled

- 2 tablespoons balsamic vinegar

- 1/4 cup pine nuts, toasted

- 1/4 cup fresh basil leaves, chopped

Preparation instructions:

1. Preheat the oven to 425°F (220°C).

2. Arrange the sliced zucchini, bell peppers, and eggplant on a large baking sheet. Drizzle with olive oil, season with salt and pepper, and toss to coat.

3. Roast for 20–25 minutes, stirring halfway, until tender and slightly browned.

4. Let cool slightly, then transfer to a serving plate.

5. Top with goat cheese, a drizzle of balsamic vinegar, toasted pine nuts, and chopped basil.

6. Serve warm or at room temperature.

Per serving: Calories: 250; Fat: 18g; Protein: 9g; Carbs: 15g; Sugar: 9g; Fiber: 5g

Difficulty rating: ★★☆☆☆

41. Chicken and Zucchini Noodles

Prep time: 20 minutes

Cook time: 10 minutes

Serves: 4

Ingredients:

- 2 large chicken breasts, thinly sliced

- 4 medium zucchinis

- 1 tablespoon garlic-infused olive oil

- Salt and pepper, to taste

- 1 teaspoon dried Italian herbs

- 1/4 cup grated Parmesan cheese (hard, aged)

- 1 tablespoon fresh basil, chopped (for garnish)

Preparation instructions:

1. Use a spiralizer to turn the zucchinis into noodles. Set aside.

2. Heat the garlic-infused olive oil in a large skillet over medium-high heat.

3. Add dried Italian herbs, salt, and pepper to the chicken slices for seasoning. Add to the skillet and heat until well cooked and golden brown, about 5 to 7 minutes. Take out and place aside the chicken from the skillet.

4. Add the zucchini noodles to the same skillet. Simmer for two to three minutes, or until somewhat soft. Take care not to overcook the noodles so they get mushy.

5. Return the cooked chicken to the skillet with the zucchini noodles. Toss to combine and heat through.

6. Serve hot, sprinkled with grated Parmesan cheese and garnished with fresh basil.

Per serving: Calories: 220; Fat: 9g; Protein: 29g; Carbs: 7g; Sugar: 4g; Fiber: 2g

Difficulty rating: ★★☆☆☆

42. *Turkey Chili*

Prep time: 20 minutes

Cook time: 40 minutes

Serves: 6

Ingredients:

- 1 tbsp garlic-infused olive oil

- 1 pound ground turkey

- 1 red bell pepper, diced

- 1 carrot, peeled and diced

- 1 zucchini, diced

- 2 tbsp tomato paste (no onion or garlic)

- 1 can (14.5 oz) diced tomatoes, no salt added

- 1 cup low-FODMAP vegetable broth

- 1 teaspoon ground cumin

- 1 teaspoon smoked paprika

- 1/2 teaspoon chili powder (adjust to taste)

- 1/2 teaspoon salt

- 1/4 teaspoon black pepper

- 1/3 cup canned black beans, rinsed and drained (approx. 120g total - optional; limit to 2 tbsp per serving)

- 1/2 cup canned corn, rinsed and drained (approx. 60g total – optional; limit to 1 tbsp per serving)

Preparation instructions:

1. In a large pot, warm garlic-infused olive oil over medium heat. Add the ground turkey and simmer for 5 to 7 minutes, or until browned and easily crumbled with a spoon.

2. Add the diced red bell pepper, carrot, and zucchini to the pot. Cook, stirring occasionally, for about 5 minutes, or until the vegetables start to soften.

3. Stir in the tomato paste, diced tomatoes, vegetable broth, cumin, smoked paprika, chili powder, salt, and black pepper. Bring the mixture to a simmer.

4. If using, add the black beans and corn to the pot. Stir well to combine.

5. Reduce the heat to low and let the chili simmer, uncovered, for 30 minutes, stirring occasionally. The chili should thicken as it cooks.

6. Taste and adjust seasoning as needed. Serve hot.

Per serving: Calories: 220; Fat: 8g; Protein: 20g; Carbs: 18g; Sugar: 6g; Fiber: 4g

Difficulty rating: ★★☆☆☆

Dinners

43. Citrus Herb Grilled Chicken

Prep time: 20 minutes

Cook time: 15 minutes

Serves: 4

Ingredients:

- 4 boneless, skinless chicken breasts
- 2 tablespoons olive oil
- 2 tablespoons lemon juice
- 1 tablespoon fresh rosemary, chopped
- 1 tablespoon fresh thyme, chopped
- 1 teaspoon salt
- 1/2 teaspoon black pepper
- Lemon slices, for garnish

Preparation instructions:

1. In a small bowl, whisk together olive oil, lemon juice, rosemary, thyme, salt, and pepper.

2. Pour the marinade over the chicken breasts that have been placed in a shallow dish. Make sure every component has a good coat. For a richer flavor, cover and chill for up to 4 hours, although at least 1 hour is preferred.

3. Preheat grill to medium-high heat. Remove chicken from marinade, discarding any excess marinade.

4. Grill chicken for 7-8 minutes on each side, or until the internal temperature reaches 165°F (74°C) and the juices run clear.

5. Remove chicken from grill and let it rest for a few minutes.

6. Serve hot, garnished with lemon slices.

Per serving: Calories: 220; Fat: 10g; Protein: 29g; Carbs: 2g; Sugar: 0g; Fiber: 0g

Difficulty rating: ★☆☆☆☆

---

44. Baked Cod with Dill

Prep time: 10 minutes

Cook time: 20 minutes

Serves: 4

Ingredients:

- 4 cod fillets (about 6 ounces each)
- 2 tablespoons olive oil
- 1/4 teaspoon salt
- 1/4 teaspoon black pepper
- 1 tablespoon fresh dill, chopped, plus extra for garnish
- 1 lemon, thinly sliced

Preparation instructions:

1. Preheat the oven to 400°F (200°C). Line a baking sheet with parchment paper.

2. Place the cod fillets on the prepared baking sheet. Brush each fillet evenly with olive oil.

3. Season the fillets with salt and black pepper. Sprinkle the chopped dill over the top of each fillet.

4. Arrange lemon slices on and around the cod fillets.

5. Bake in the preheated oven for 18-20 minutes, or until the fish flakes easily with a fork.

6. Garnish with additional fresh dill before serving.

Per serving: Calories: 190; Fat: 7g; Protein: 30g; Carbs: 2g; Sugar: 0g; Fiber: 0g

Difficulty rating: ★☆☆☆☆

---

45. Herb-Crusted Chicken with Roasted Vegetables

Prep time: 15 minutes

Cook time: 35 minutes

Serves: 4

Ingredients:

- 4 boneless, skinless chicken breasts
- 1 tablespoon garlic-infused olive oil
- 1 tablespoon fresh thyme, chopped
- 1 tablespoon fresh rosemary, chopped
- 1 teaspoon dried oregano
- 1 teaspoon dried basil
- 1/2 teaspoon salt
- 1/4 teaspoon ground black pepper
- 1 large zucchini, sliced
- 1 large carrot, sliced
- 1 red bell pepper, sliced
- 1 yellow bell pepper, sliced

Preparation instructions:

1. Preheat your oven to 400°F (200°C).

2. In a small bowl, combine the garlic-infused olive oil, thyme, rosemary, oregano, basil, salt, and pepper.

3. Coat the chicken breasts thoroughly by rubbing them with the herb mixture.

4. Place the chicken breasts on a baking sheet lined with parchment paper.

5. Around the chicken on the baking sheet, arrange the sliced bell peppers, carrots, and zucchini.

6. Drizzle a little more garlic-infused olive oil over the vegetables and season with additional salt and pepper.

7. Roast in the preheated oven for 25-30 minutes, or until the chicken is cooked through and the vegetables are tender.

8. Serve hot and enjoy a balanced, nutritious dinner.

Per serving: Calories: 320; Fat: 14g; Protein: 30g; Carbs: 15g; Sugar: 6g; Fiber: 4g

Difficulty rating: ★★☆☆☆

---

46. Quinoa Stuffed Bell Peppers

Prep time: 25 minutes

Cook time: 35 minutes

Serves: 4

Ingredients:

- 4 large bell peppers, any color
- 1 cup quinoa, rinsed
- 2 cups low-FODMAP vegetable broth
- 1 tablespoon garlic-infused olive oil
- 1 cup spinach, chopped
- 1/2 cup carrots, grated
- 1/2 cup zucchini, diced
- 1/4 cup fresh basil, chopped
- 1 teaspoon dried oregano
- Salt and pepper, to taste
- 1/2 cup grated cheddar cheese (lactose-free if necessary)

Directions:

1. Preheat the oven to 375°F (190°C).

2. Slice off the bell peppers' tops, then take out the seeds and membranes. Put aside.

3. Heat the vegetable broth in a medium saucepan until it begins to boil. After adding the quinoa, turn down the heat to low, cover, and simmer until the liquid is completely absorbed—about 15 minutes. After turning off the heat, leave it for five minutes. Using a fork, fluff.

4. Heat the garlic-infused oil in a skillet over medium heat. Add the spinach, carrots, and zucchini. Cook for 5-7 minutes, or until the vegetables are tender.

5. Combine the cooked quinoa with the sautéed vegetables, fresh basil, oregano, salt, and pepper in a large bowl. Mix well.

6. Tightly stuff the quinoa mixture within the bell peppers.

7. Transfer the filled peppers into a baking dish and tent-like cover with aluminum foil.

8. Bake for twenty-five minutes. Take off the foil, add some grated cheese to the peppers' tops, and bake for a further ten minutes, or until the cheese is bubbling and melted.

9. Serve hot.

Per serving: Calories: 320; Fat: 12g; Protein: 12g; Carbs: 44g; Sugar: 8g; Fiber: 7g

Difficulty rating: ★★☆☆

47. Lemon Shrimp Skewers

Prep time: 20 minutes

Cook time: 10 minutes

Serves: 4

Ingredients:

- 1 pound large shrimp, peeled and deveined
- 2 tablespoons garlic-infused olive oil
- Juice of 1 lemon
- 1 tablespoon fresh parsley, finely chopped
- Salt and pepper, to taste
- 8 bamboo skewers, soaked in water for 30 minutes

Directions:

1. In a large bowl, combine the shrimp, garlic-infused olive oil, lemon juice, parsley, salt, and pepper. Toss to coat the shrimp evenly.

2. Preheat your grill to medium-high heat.

3. Put the shrimp on the bamboo skewers that have been soaked.

4. Grill the skewers for 2-3 minutes on each side or until the shrimp turn pink and opaque.

5. Serve immediately, garnished with additional parsley if desired.

Per serving: Calories: 180; Fat: 7g; Protein: 24g; Carbs: 2g; Sugar: 0g; Fiber: 0g

Difficulty rating: ★☆☆☆☆

48. Beef and Vegetable Stir-Fry

Prep time: 20 minutes

Cook time: 15 minutes

Serves: 4

Ingredients:

- 1 lb beef sirloin, thinly sliced
- 2 tbsp garlic-infused olive oil
- 1 cup broccoli florets
- 1 cup sliced carrots
- 1 red bell pepper, sliced
- 1 tbsp soy sauce (gluten-free, low-sodium)
- 1 tbsp oyster sauce (check for low-FODMAP certification)
- 1 teaspoon sesame oil
- 1/2 teaspoon ground ginger
- 1/4 cup water
- Salt and pepper, to taste

Preparation instructions:

1. Heat 1 tablespoon of garlic-infused olive oil in a large skillet or wok over medium-high heat.

2. Add the beef slices to the skillet and stir-fry for 2-3 minutes until browned. Remove beef from skillet and set aside.

3. Transfer the remaining tablespoon of garlic-infused olive oil to the same skillet. Add the red bell pepper, carrots, and broccoli. Stir-fry the vegetables for five to seven minutes, or until they are crisp but soft.

4. In a small bowl, whisk together the low-sodium soy sauce, oyster sauce, sesame oil, ground ginger, and water.

5. Place the steak back in the skillet along with the veggies. Cover the beef and vegetables with the sauce mixture. Cook, stirring constantly, for an additional two to three minutes, or until everything is well cooked and covered with sauce. To taste, add salt and pepper for seasoning. Serve hot.

Per serving: Calories: 280; Fat: 14g; Protein: 26g; Carbs: 12g; Sugar: 5g; Fiber: 3g

Difficulty rating: ★★☆☆☆

---

49. Chicken and Broccoli Casserole

Prep time: 20 minutes

Cook time: 35 minutes

Serves: 4

Ingredients:

- 2 cups broccoli florets

- 1 lb chicken breast, cubed

- 1 tablespoon garlic-infused olive oil

- 1 cup lactose-free milk

- 2 tablespoons gluten-free all-purpose flour

- 1 cup grated cheddar cheese (lactose-free)

- 1/2 teaspoon salt

- 1/4 teaspoon black pepper

- 1/4 teaspoon paprika

- 1/2 cup gluten-free breadcrumbs

- 1 tablespoon melted unsalted butter (lactose-free)

Preparation instructions:

1. Preheat the oven to 375°F (190°C). Lightly grease a 9x13 inch baking dish.

2. Steam the broccoli florets until just tender, about 3-4 minutes, then spread them out in the bottom of the prepared baking dish.

3. In a skillet over medium heat, cook the cubed chicken in garlic-infused olive oil until browned and no longer pink inside, about 5-7 minutes. Spread the cooked chicken over the broccoli.

4. Combine gluten-free flour and lactose-free milk in the same skillet and mix over medium heat until smooth. Cook until the sauce thickens, about 2 to 3 minutes. Take off the heat and mix in the melted cheddar cheese after grating. Add paprika, salt, and pepper for seasoning.

5. Evenly cover the chicken and broccoli in the baking dish with the cheese sauce.

6. In a small bowl, mix together gluten-free breadcrumbs and melted butter. Sprinkle this mixture over the top of the casserole.

7. Bake for 25 minutes in a preheated oven, or until the casserole is bubbling and the breadcrumb coating is golden brown.

8. Let the casserole cool for 5 minutes before serving.

Per serving: Calories: 450; Fat: 22g; Protein: 38g; Carbs: 25g; Sugar: 5g; Fiber: 3g

Difficulty rating: ★★☆☆☆

50. Turkey Meatballs with Zucchini Noodles

Prep time: 25 minutes

Cook time: 15 minutes

Serves: 4

Ingredients:

- 1 lb ground turkey
- 1/4 cup gluten-free breadcrumbs
- 1/4 cup grated Parmesan cheese (hard, aged)
- 1 large egg
- 1 tablespoon garlic-infused olive oil
- 1 teaspoon dried oregano
- 1/2 teaspoon salt
- 1/4 teaspoon black pepper
- 4 medium zucchinis
- 1 tablespoon olive oil
- Salt and pepper, to taste

Directions:

1. Ground turkey, gluten-free breadcrumbs, egg, grated Parmesan cheese, garlic-infused olive oil, dried oregano, salt, and black pepper should all be combined in a big bowl. Blend thoroughly until all components are dispersed equally.

2. Form the mixture into 16 meatballs, approximately 1 inch in diameter.

3. Heat a large skillet over medium heat and add the meatballs. Cook for 8-10 minutes, turning occasionally, until browned on all sides and cooked through. Remove from skillet and set aside.

4. To make noodles out of the zucchini, use a spiralizer. To make thin ribbons without a spiralizer, use a vegetable peeler.

5. Add 1 tablespoon of olive oil to the same skillet you used to cook the meatballs and place over medium heat. Season with salt and pepper, add the zucchini noodles, and sauté for two to three minutes, or until they are just soft.

6. Divide the zucchini noodles among plates and top with turkey meatballs.

Per serving: Calories: 320; Fat: 18g; Protein: 28g; Carbs: 12g; Sugar: 5g; Fiber: 3g

Difficulty rating: ★★☆☆☆

---

51. Salmon with Zucchini and Lemon Dill

Prep time: 15 minutes

Cook time: 20 minutes

Serves: 4

Ingredients:

- 4 salmon fillets (6 ounces each)
- 1 cup canned bamboo shoots, drained and rinsed
- 3/4 pound zucchini, sliced (approx. 2 cups)
- 2 tablespoons garlic-infused olive oil
- Salt and pepper, to taste
- 1 lemon, thinly sliced
- 1 tablespoon fresh dill, chopped

Directions:

1. Preheat the oven to 400°F (200°C) and line a large baking sheet with parchment paper.

2. Arrange the salmon fillets on one side of the sheet and the sliced zucchini and bamboo shoots on the other.

3. Drizzle everything with garlic-infused olive oil and season with salt and pepper to taste.

4. Top each salmon fillet with a lemon slice or two.

5. Bake in the preheated oven for 18–20 minutes, or until the salmon flakes easily with a fork and the vegetables are tender.

6. Sprinkle with fresh dill and serve immediately.

Per serving: Calories: 340; Fat: 22g; Protein: 34g; Carbs: 5g; Sugar: 2g; Fiber: 2g

Difficulty rating: ★☆☆☆☆

---

52. Vegetable Paella

Prep time: 20 minutes

Cook time: 35 minutes

Serves: 4

Ingredients:

- 1 cup low-FODMAP vegetable broth

- 1/2 cup quinoa

- 1 tablespoon garlic-infused olive oil

- 1 red bell pepper, diced

- 1 medium carrot, diced

- 1 zucchini, diced

- 1/2 cup green beans, trimmed and cut into 1-inch pieces

- 1/2 teaspoon saffron threads

- 1 teaspoon smoked paprika

- 1/2 teaspoon salt

- 1/4 teaspoon black pepper

- 1/4 cup chopped fresh parsley

- Lemon wedges, for serving

Preparation instructions:

1. Bring the low-FODMAP vegetable broth to a boil in a small saucepan. After adding the quinoa, turn down the heat to low, cover, and simmer until the liquid is completely absorbed—about 15 minutes. Take it off the fire and leave it for five minutes before fluffing it with a fork.

2. While the quinoa is cooking, heat the garlic-infused olive oil in a large skillet over medium heat. Add the red bell pepper, carrot, and zucchini. Cook for 5-7 minutes, or until the vegetables are just tender.

3. Stir in the green beans, saffron threads, smoked paprika, salt, and black pepper. Cook for an additional 2 minutes.

4. Add the cooked quinoa to the skillet with the vegetables. Stir well to combine and cook for another 5 minutes, or until everything is heated through.

5. Remove from heat and stir in the chopped parsley.

6. Serve the vegetable paella with lemon wedges on the side.

Per serving: Calories: 190; Fat: 5g; Protein: 6g; Carbs: 30g; Sugar: 5g; Fiber: 6g

Difficulty rating: ★★☆☆☆

53. Herb-Roasted Pork and Vegetables

Prep time: 20 minutes

Cook time: 40 minutes

Serves: 4

Ingredients:

- 1 (1.5-pound) pork tenderloin
- 2 tablespoons olive oil, divided
- 1 teaspoon salt, divided
- 1/2 teaspoon black pepper, divided
- 1/2 teaspoon dried rosemary
- 1/2 teaspoon dried thyme
- 2 medium carrots, peeled and sliced
- 2 medium parsnips, peeled and sliced
- 1 small butternut squash, peeled, seeded, and cubed
- 1 tablespoon garlic-infused olive oil
- 1 tablespoon balsamic vinegar

Directions:

1. Preheat the oven to 400°F (200°C).

2. Rub the pork tenderloin with 1 tablespoon of olive oil, 1/2 teaspoon salt, 1/4 teaspoon black pepper, rosemary, and thyme. Place in a roasting pan.

3. In a large bowl, toss the carrots, parsnips, and butternut squash with the remaining olive oil, garlic-infused olive oil, balsamic vinegar, and the remaining salt and pepper until well coated.

4. Arrange the vegetables around the pork in the roasting pan.

5. Roast in the preheated oven for 25 minutes. Remove the pan from the oven and stir the vegetables.

6. Return the pan to the oven and continue roasting until the pork reaches an internal temperature of 145°F (63°C) and the vegetables are tender, about 15 more minutes.

7. Let the pork rest for 5 minutes before slicing. Serve the sliced pork tenderloin with the roasted vegetables.

Per serving: Calories: 380; Fat: 15g; Protein: 35g; Carbs: 29g; Sugar: 7g; Fiber: 6g

Difficulty rating: ★★☆☆☆

54. Lentil and Vegetable Stew

Prep time: 20 minutes

Cook time: 40 minutes

Serves: 6

Ingredients:

- 1 tablespoon garlic-infused olive oil

- 1 cup diced carrots

- 1 cup diced celery

- 1 cup diced red bell pepper

- 1 cup dried red lentils, rinsed (use no more than ½ cup cooked lentils per serving to remain low-FODMAP)

- 1 can (14.5 oz) diced tomatoes, no salt added

- 4 cups low-FODMAP vegetable broth

- 1 teaspoon dried thyme

- 1 teaspoon dried rosemary

- Salt and pepper, to taste

- 2 cups chopped spinach

Directions:

1. In a big pot, warm the garlic-infused olive oil over medium heat. Add the red bell pepper, celery, and carrots and sauté for 5 to 6 minutes, or until the veggies begin to soften and become fragrant.

2. Stir in the red lentils, diced tomatoes, and vegetable broth. Season with thyme, rosemary, salt, and pepper.

3. Bring the mixture to a boil, then reduce the heat to low and simmer, covered, for 30 minutes, or until the lentils are tender.

4. Add the chopped spinach to the pot and cook for an additional 5 minutes, or until the spinach has wilted.

5. If necessary, add more salt and pepper to taste the food. Serve hot.

Per serving: Calories: 210; Fat: 3g; Protein: 12g; Carbs: 35g; Sugar: 6g; Fiber: 15g

Difficulty rating: ★★☆☆☆

55. Chicken Fajita Bowls

Prep time: 20 minutes

Cook time: 15 minutes

Serves: 4

Ingredients:

- 1 lb chicken breast, thinly sliced
- 2 tablespoons garlic-infused olive oil, divided
- 1 teaspoon cumin
- 1 teaspoon paprika
- Salt and pepper, to taste
- 1 red bell pepper, sliced
- 1 green bell pepper, sliced
- 1 yellow bell pepper, sliced
- 4 cups cooked brown rice, cooled
- 1/4 cup fresh cilantro, chopped
- 1 lime, cut into wedges
- 1/4 cup lactose-free sour cream (optional)

Directions:

1. In a bowl, toss chicken with 1 tbsp garlic-infused olive oil, cumin, paprika, salt, and pepper.

2. Heat a large skillet over medium-high. Cook chicken for 5–7 minutes until cooked through. Remove and set aside.

3. In the same skillet, add remaining 1 tbsp oil and sauté bell peppers for about 5 minutes until tender-crisp..

4. Return the cooked chicken to the skillet with the peppers and stir to combine. Cook for an additional 2 minutes to reheat the chicken.

5. Divide the cooked brown rice among four bowls. Top each bowl with the chicken and pepper mixture.

6. Garnish each bowl with chopped cilantro, a wedge of lime, and a dollop of lactose-free sour cream, if using.

7. Serve immediately.

Per serving: Calories: 350; Fat: 9g; Protein: 28g; Carbs: 40g; Sugar: 3g; Fiber: 5g

Difficulty rating: ★★☆☆☆

56. Spaghetti Squash with Marinara

Prep time: 15 minutes

Cook time: 45 minutes

Serves: 4

Ingredients:

- 1 medium spaghetti squash

- 2 tablespoons olive oil

- Salt and pepper, to taste

- 1 cup low-FODMAP marinara sauce (ensure no onion or garlic)

- 1/4 cup fresh basil, chopped

- 1/2 cup grated Parmesan cheese (hard, aged)

Directions:

1. Preheat the oven to 400°F (200°C). Line a baking sheet with parchment paper.

2. Scoop out the seeds after cutting the spaghetti squash in half lengthwise. Season with salt and pepper and drizzle one tablespoon of olive oil inside each half.

3. On the baking sheet that has been prepared, place the squash halves cut-side down. Roast for 30 to 40 minutes in a preheated oven, or until the meat is fork-tender and easily shreds.

4. While the squash is roasting, warm the marinara sauce in a small saucepan over medium heat.

5. When the squash is cooked through, allow it to cool for a few minutes before handling. To make spaghetti-like strands, scrape the insides of the squash with a fork.

6. Divide the squash strands among 4 plates. Top each serving with warm marinara sauce.

7. Garnish with fresh basil and grated Parmesan cheese before serving.

Per serving: Calories: 210; Fat: 11g; Protein: 7g; Carbs: 23g; Sugar: 8g; Fiber: 5g

Difficulty rating: ★★☆☆☆

57. Tofu and Vegetable Stir-Fry

Prep time: 15 minutes

Cook time: 10 minutes

Serves: 4

Ingredients:

- 14 oz firm tofu, pressed and cut into cubes

- 2 tbsp garlic-infused olive oil

- 1 cup carrots, thinly sliced

- 1 cup bell peppers (red and yellow), sliced

- 1 cup broccoli florets

- 1 cup green beans, trimmed (limit to 75g or ½ cup per person)

- 2 tbsp soy sauce (gluten-free, low-sodium)

- 1 tbsp ginger, grated

- 1 tbsp rice vinegar

- 1 tbsp maple syrup

- 1 teaspoon sesame oil

- Salt and pepper, to taste

- Sesame seeds, for garnish

- Green onions (green parts only), sliced for garnish

Directions:

1. Heat the garlic-infused olive oil in a large skillet or wok over medium-high heat.

2. Add the tofu cubes to the skillet and fry for 4-5 minutes, or until golden brown on all sides. Remove tofu from the skillet and set aside.

3. In the same skillet, add another tablespoon of garlic-infused olive oil if needed. Add the carrots, bell peppers, broccoli, and green beans. Stir-fry for 3-4 minutes, or until vegetables are tender but still crisp.

4. In a small bowl, whisk together the low-sodium soy sauce, grated ginger, rice vinegar, maple syrup, and sesame oil. Pour this sauce over the cooked vegetables in the skillet.

5. Return the tofu to the skillet. Toss everything together and cook for another 2 minutes, allowing the tofu to absorb the flavors of the sauce.

6. Season with salt and pepper to taste.

7. Serve hot, garnished with sesame seeds and sliced green onions.

Per serving: Calories: 220; Fat: 12g; Protein: 13g; Carbs: 18g; Sugar: 7g; Fiber: 4g

Difficulty rating: ★★☆☆☆

Quick Vegetarian and Vegan Recipes

Prep time: 15 minutes

Cook time: 10 minutes

Serves: 4

Ingredients:

- 1 zucchini, cut into 1/2-inch slices

- 1 yellow squash, cut into 1/2-inch slices

- 1 red bell pepper, cut into 1-inch pieces

- 1 green bell pepper, cut into 1-inch pieces

- 8 cherry tomatoes

- 8 button mushrooms, stems removed

- 1/4 cup garlic-infused olive oil

- Salt and pepper, to taste

- 2 tablespoons balsamic vinegar

- 1 teaspoon dried Italian herbs

Preparation instructions:

1. Preheat the grill to medium-high heat.

2. Thread the zucchini, yellow squash, red bell pepper, green bell pepper, cherry tomatoes, and mushrooms alternately onto skewers.

3. In a small bowl, whisk together the garlic-infused olive oil, balsamic vinegar, and dried Italian herbs.

4. Brush the vegetable skewers with the olive oil mixture and season with salt and pepper.

5. For around ten minutes, or until the veggies are soft and lightly browned, grill the skewers, rotating them from time to time.

6. Remove from grill and serve immediately.

Per serving: Calories: 120; Fat: 7g; Protein: 2g; Carbs: 13g; Sugar: 7g; Fiber: 3g

Difficulty rating: ★ ☆ ☆ ☆ ☆

Prep time: 20 minutes

Cook time: 10 minutes

Serves: 4

Ingredients:

- 1 cup dried green lentils, rinsed

- 2 cups water

- 1 tablespoon garlic-infused olive oil

- 1 teaspoon ground cumin

- 1 teaspoon smoked paprika

- 1/2 teaspoon chili powder

- Salt and pepper, to taste

- 8 gluten-free corn tortillas

- 1 cup lettuce, shredded

- 1 large tomato, diced

- 1/2 cup cucumber, diced

- 1/4 cup red cabbage, shredded

- 1/4 cup carrots, shredded

- 1/4 cup fresh cilantro, chopped

Preparation instructions:

1. Heat the two cups of water in a medium-sized saucepan until it boils. Once the lentils are soft and the water has been absorbed, add the lentils, lower the heat to low, cover, and simmer for 25 to 30 minutes. Remove any extra water.

2. Heat the garlic-infused olive oil in a skillet over medium heat. Add the cooked lentils, cumin, smoked paprika, chili powder, salt, and pepper. Cook for 5 minutes, stirring frequently, until the lentils are well coated with the spices.

3. In a dry skillet over medium heat, reheat the corn tortillas for about 30 seconds on each side, or until they become soft and malleable.

4. To assemble the tacos, divide the spiced lentil mixture evenly among the tortillas. Top each taco with lettuce, tomato, cucumber, red cabbage, carrots, and cilantro.

5. Serve immediately.

Per serving: Calories: 300; Fat:7g; Protein: 13g; Carbs: 47g; Sugar: 4g; Fiber: 13g

Difficulty rating: ★★☆☆☆

---

60. Stuffed Zucchini Boats

Prep time: 20 minutes

Cook time: 30 minutes

Serves: 4

Ingredients:

- 4 medium zucchinis

- 1 cup cooked quinoa

- 1/2 cup bell peppers, finely diced

- 1/2 cup carrots, shredded

- 1/4 cup sun-dried tomatoes, chopped

- 1/4 cup olives, sliced

- 1/4 cup feta cheese, crumbled (use vegan feta for a vegan version)

- 2 tablespoons pine nuts

- 1 tablespoon olive oil

- 1 teaspoon dried oregano

- Salt and pepper, to taste

- Fresh basil, for garnish

Preparation instructions:

1. Preheat the oven to 375°F (190°C). Line a baking sheet with parchment paper.

2. Cut the zucchinis in half lengthwise and scoop out the insides with a spoon, leaving about 1/4 inch of flesh on the skin to form boats.

3. In a large bowl, combine the cooked quinoa, bell peppers, carrots, sun-dried tomatoes, olives, feta cheese, pine nuts, olive oil, and dried oregano. Season with salt and pepper to taste.

4. Stuff the quinoa mixture into the hollowed-out zucchini boats, pressing down gently to pack the filling.

5. Once the baking sheet is ready, place the filled zucchini boats on it. Bake for 25 to 30 minutes, or until the filling is heated through and the zucchinis are soft.

6. Garnish with fresh basil before serving.

Per serving: Calories: 220; Fat: 10g; Protein: 8g; Carbs: 27g; Sugar: 8g; Fiber: 5g

Difficulty rating: ★★☆☆☆

61. Vegetarian Chili

Prep time: 20 minutes

Cook time: 30 minutes

Serves: 6

Ingredients:

- 1 tablespoon olive oil

- 1 large carrot, peeled and diced

- 1 red bell pepper, diced

- 1 green bell pepper, diced

- 1 zucchini, diced

- 1 cup (240g) canned black beans, rinsed and drained (approx. 40g per serving)

- 1½ cups (450g) canned green beans, rinsed and drained (limit to 75g per serving)

- 1 can (15 oz) diced tomatoes, with juice

- 2 cups vegetable broth, low-FODMAP certified

- 1 teaspoon ground cumin

- 1 teaspoon smoked paprika

- 1/2 teaspoon chili powder (adjust to taste)

- Salt and pepper, to taste

- Fresh cilantro, chopped (for garnish)

Preparation instructions:

1. In a big pot, warm the olive oil over medium heat. Add the zucchini, red, green, and carrot bell peppers. Cook the veggies for 5 to 7 minutes, or until they become tender.

2. Add measured black beans, green beans, diced tomatoes with their juice, and vegetable broth to the pot. Stir well to combine.

3. Season with ground cumin, smoked paprika, chili powder, salt, and pepper. Stir again to distribute the spices evenly.

4. Bring the mixture to a boil, then reduce the heat to low and simmer, uncovered, for 20 minutes, stirring occasionally.

5. Taste and adjust the seasoning if necessary. If the chili is too thick, add a little more vegetable broth to reach your desired consistency.

6. Serve hot, garnished with fresh cilantro.

Per serving: Calories: 200; Fat: 3g; Protein: 10g; Carbs: 33g; Sugar: 5g; Fiber: 10g

Difficulty rating: ★★☆☆☆

62. Vegan Buddha Bowl

Prep time: 20 minutes

Cook time: 0 minutes

Serves: 4

Ingredients:

- 2 cups cooked quinoa

- 1 cup shredded purple cabbage

- 1 cup sliced cucumber

- 1 cup shredded carrots

- 1 cup diced red bell pepper

- 1/2 cup boiled edamame (Low-FODMAP portion)

- 1/4 cup sliced green onions (green parts only)

- 2 tablespoons sesame seeds

For the dressing:

- 1/4 cup low-FODMAP peanut or almond butter

- 2 tablespoons tamari sauce (gluten-free)

- 1 tablespoon maple syrup

- 1 tablespoon rice vinegar

- 1 tablespoon sesame oil

- 1/4 cup water (to thin the dressing)

- Salt and pepper, to taste

Preparation instructions:

1. Divide the cooked quinoa among four bowls.

2. Arrange the purple cabbage, cucumber, carrots, red bell pepper, and edamame on top of the quinoa in each bowl.

3. Sprinkle sliced green onions and sesame seeds over each bowl.

4. In a small bowl, whisk together the peanut or almond butter, tamari sauce, maple syrup, rice vinegar, sesame oil, and water until smooth and well combined. Season with salt and pepper to taste.

5. Drizzle the dressing over each bowl before serving.

Per serving: Calories: 360; Fat: 19g; Protein: 12g; Carbs: 35g; Sugar: 7g; Fiber: 8g

Difficulty rating: ★★☆☆☆

Allergen information: Gluten-free, Dairy-free, Nut-free option (if using sunflower seed butter instead of peanut or almond butter), Vegan

---

63. Vegetarian Stuffed Peppers

Prep time: 20 minutes

Cook time: 35 minutes

Serves: 4

Ingredients:

- 4 large bell peppers, tops cut away and seeds removed

- 1 tablespoon garlic-infused olive oil

- 1 cup quinoa, rinsed

- 2 cups low-FODMAP vegetable broth

- 2/3 cup canned black beans, rinsed and drained (160g total / 40g per serving)

- 1/2 cup corn kernels (fresh or frozen) (120g total / 30g per serving)

- 1 teaspoon ground cumin

- 1/2 teaspoon chili powder

- 1/2 cup grated cheddar cheese (lactose-free if necessary)

- 1/4 cup chopped fresh cilantro, plus extra for garnish

- Salt and pepper, to taste

Preparation instructions:

1. Turn the oven on to 375°F, or 190°C. Place the bell peppers cut-side up in a baking dish.

2. In a medium saucepan, heat the garlic-infused olive oil over medium heat. Add the quinoa and toast for 2-3 minutes, stirring frequently.

3. After adding the low-FODMAP vegetable broth, heat it until it boils. For fifteen to twenty minutes, or when the quinoa is soft and the liquid has been absorbed, reduce heat to low, cover, and simmer.

4. Stir in the black beans, corn, cumin, chili powder, half of the cheddar cheese, and chopped cilantro. Season with salt and pepper to taste.

5. Pack the bell peppers firmly with the quinoa mixture by spooning it inside and pressing down. Place the remaining cheddar cheese on top.

6. Cover the baking dish with aluminum foil and bake for 25 minutes. Remove the foil and bake for an additional 10 minutes, or until the cheese is bubbly and the peppers are tender.

7. Garnish with additional chopped cilantro before serving.

Per serving: Calories: 305; Fat: 8g; Protein: 14g; Carbs: 41g; Sugar: 6g; Fiber: 8g

---

64. Vegan Quinoa Salad

Prep time: 20 minutes

Cook time: 0 minutes

Serves: 4

Ingredients:

- 1 cup quinoa, rinsed

- 2 cups water

- 1/2 cup cucumber, diced

- 1/2 cup red bell pepper, diced

- 1/4 cup Kalamata olives, sliced

- 1/2 cup green onions (green parts only), finely chopped

- 1/4 cup cherry tomatoes, halved

- 1/4 cup fresh parsley, chopped

- 1/4 cup fresh mint, chopped

- 2 tablespoons olive oil

- 2 tablespoons lemon juice

- Salt and pepper, to taste

- Optional: 1/2 avocado, diced (limit to 30g per serving if sensitive)

Preparation instructions:

1. In a medium saucepan, bring 2 cups of water to a boil. Add quinoa, reduce heat to low, cover, and simmer for 15 minutes or until all the water is absorbed. Remove from heat and let it stand covered for 5 minutes. Fluff with a fork and allow to cool.

2. In a large bowl, combine cooled quinoa, cucumber, red bell pepper, Kalamata olives, green onion, cherry tomatoes, parsley, and mint.

3. In a small bowl, whisk together olive oil and lemon juice. Pour over the quinoa mixture and toss to coat. Season with salt and pepper to taste.

4. Gently fold in the diced avocado if using.

5. Serve chilled or at room temperature.

Per serving: Calories: 310:; Fat: 15g; Protein: 8g; Carbs: 38g; Sugar: 3g; Fiber: 7g

65. Vegetarian Sushi Rolls

Prep time: 30 minutes

Cook time: 0 minutes

Serves: 4

Ingredients:

- 1 cup sushi rice, rinsed and cooked according to package instructions, then cooled

- 4 sheets nori (seaweed)

- 1/2 cucumber, julienned

- 1 carrot, peeled and julienned

- optional: 1/2 avocado, sliced (use a maximum of 30g per serving)

- 1/2 red bell pepper, julienned

- 1/4 cup pickled radish, optional

- 2 tablespoons low-FODMAP soy sauce or tamari for dipping

- Wasabi, to taste (optional)

- Pickled ginger, for serving

Preparation instructions:

1. Arrange a nori sheet on a piece of parchment paper or a bamboo sushi mat.

2. Spread about 1/4 of the cooked rice evenly over the nori, leaving a small margin at the top edge. Wet your hands to prevent sticking.

3. Arrange a few pieces of cucumber, carrot, avocado (if using), red bell pepper, and pickled radish (if using) in a line across the rice, about one-third of the way up from the bottom.

4. To begin making the sushi roll, gently pull the edge of the mat or paper nearest you and roll it over the ingredients. As you proceed, firmly press the roll together using the mat or paper.

5. Continue rolling until you reach the end of the nori, wetting the exposed margin slightly to seal the roll.

6. Cut the roll into six to eight pieces using a sharp, moist knife. Continue using the remaining ingredients to create a total of four rolls.

7. Serve the vegetarian sushi rolls with low-FODMAP soy sauce or tamari, wasabi, and pickled ginger on the side.

Per serving: Calories: 210; Fat: 7g; Protein: 4g; Carbs: 34g; Sugar: 3g; Fiber: 5g

Difficulty rating: ★★☆☆☆

Allergen information: Gluten-free (if using gluten-free soy sauce or tamari), Nut-free, Dairy-free, Vegan.

66. Vegan Black Bean Burgers

Prep time: 20 minutes

Cook time: 10 minutes

Serves: 4

Ingredients:

- 2/3 cup canned black beans, rinsed and drained (160g total / 40g per serving)

- 1/2 cup quinoa, cooked

- 1/4 cup red bell pepper, finely chopped

- 1/2 cup green onions (green parts only), finely chopped

- 1/4 cup cilantro, chopped

- 1 teaspoon cumin

- 1/2 teaspoon smoked paprika

- Salt and pepper, to taste

- 1 flax egg (3 tbsp of water and one tbsp of ground flaxseed combined; let lie for fifteen minutes)

- 1/2 cup gluten-free breadcrumbs

- 2 tablespoons olive oil, for frying

Preparation instructions:

1. In a large bowl, mash the black beans with a fork or potato masher until mostly smooth.

2. Add the cooked quinoa, red bell pepper, green onion, cilantro, cumin, smoked paprika, salt, pepper, flax egg, and breadcrumbs to the mashed beans. Stir until well combined.

3. Form the mixture into 4 equal-sized patties.

4. Heat the olive oil in a large skillet over medium heat. Place the patties in the skillet and cook for about 5 minutes on each side, or until they are golden brown and heated through.

Per serving: Calories: 260; Fat: 9g; Protein: 9g; Carbs: 37g; Sugar: 2g; Fiber: 8g

Difficulty rating: ★★☆☆

---

67. Vegetarian Pad Thai

Prep time: 20 minutes

Cook time: 10 minutes

Serves: 4

Ingredients:

- 8 oz rice noodles

- 1/4 cup low-sodium soy sauce (ensure gluten-free for a fully low-FODMAP meal)

- 2 tablespoons maple syrup

- 1 tablespoon rice vinegar

- 1 tablespoon lime juice

- 1 tablespoon garlic-infused olive oil

- 1 cup firm tofu, cubed

- 1 cup carrots, julienned

- 1 cup red bell pepper, thinly sliced

- 1/2 cup green onions (green parts only), chopped

- 1/4 cup peanuts, chopped

- 1/4 cup fresh cilantro, chopped

- Lime wedges, for serving

Preparation instructions:

1. Cook rice noodles according to package instructions, then drain and set aside.

2. In a small bowl, whisk together soy sauce, maple syrup, rice vinegar, and lime juice. Set aside.

3. Heat garlic-infused olive oil in a large skillet over medium heat. Add tofu cubes and cook until golden brown on all sides, about 5-7 minutes. Remove tofu from skillet and set aside.

4. In the same skillet, add carrots and red bell pepper. Stir-fry for 2-3 minutes until just tender.

5. Add the cooked noodles, tofu, and soy sauce mixture to the skillet. Toss everything together and cook for an additional 2-3 minutes, until heated through.

6. Remove from heat and stir in green onions, peanuts, and cilantro.

7. Serve hot, garnished with lime wedges.

Per serving: Calories: 350; Fat: 9g; Protein: 12g; Carbs: 56g; Sugar: 8g; Fiber: 3g

Difficulty rating: ★★★☆☆

---

68. Vegan Stuffed Zucchini Cups

Prep time: 20 minutes

Cook time: 25 minutes

Serves: 4

Ingredients:

- 2 large zucchinis, cut into 2-inch thick rounds and scooped to create cups
- 1 tablespoon garlic-infused olive oil
- 1/2 cup quinoa, cooked
- 1/4 cup walnuts, chopped
- 1/4 cup nutritional yeast
- 1/4 cup fresh parsley, chopped
- 1/4 teaspoon smoked paprika
- Salt and pepper, to taste
- 1 tablespoon lemon juice
- 1/4 cup gluten-free breadcrumbs

Preparation instructions:

1. Preheat the oven to 375°F (190°C) and line a baking sheet with parchment paper.

2. Using a small spoon or melon baller, gently scoop out the centers of each zucchini round to create small "cups."

3. In a skillet over medium heat, warm the garlic-infused olive oil. Add the scooped-out zucchini flesh (optional, for moisture and flavor) and cook for 3–4 minutes until soft.

4. In a large bowl, combine the cooked zucchini, quinoa, walnuts, nutritional yeast, parsley, smoked paprika, salt, pepper, and lemon juice. Mix thoroughly.

5. Spoon the mixture into each zucchini cup, pressing down lightly to pack.

6. Sprinkle the gluten-free breadcrumbs over the tops.

7. Bake for 25 minutes, or until golden on top and zucchini is tender.

8. Serve warm.

Per serving: Calories: 170; Fat: 9g; Protein: 7g; Carbs: 16g; Sugar: 2g; Fiber: 3g

Difficulty rating: ★★☆☆☆

Allergen information: Gluten-free, Dairy-free, Vegan.

69. Vegetarian Lasagna

Prep time: 25 minutes

Cook time: 45 minutes

Serves: 6

Ingredients:

- 9 gluten-free lasagna noodles

- 2 tablespoons garlic-infused olive oil

- 1 cup diced zucchini

- 1 cup diced bell pepper

- 1 cup shredded carrots

- 1 cup chopped spinach

- 2 cups crushed tomatoes (no onion or garlic)

- 1 teaspoon dried basil

- 1 teaspoon dried oregano

- Salt and pepper, to taste

- 1 1/2 cups lactose-free ricotta cheese (divided into 6 servings = 1/4 cup per person, within low-FODMAP limit)

- 1 egg

- 2 cups lactose-free shredded mozzarella cheese (about 1/3 cup per serving)

- 1/2 cup grated Parmesan cheese (hard, aged)

Preparation instructions:

1. Preheat the oven to 375°F (190°C). Cook the gluten-free lasagna noodles according to package instructions; drain and set aside.

2. Heat the garlic-infused olive oil in a large skillet over medium heat. Add zucchini, bell pepper, and carrots. Cook for 5-7 minutes until vegetables are tender. Cook the chopped spinach until it wilts after adding it.

3. Stir in crushed tomatoes, basil, oregano, salt, and pepper. Simmer for 10 minutes.

4. Combine the egg and lactose-free ricotta cheese in a bowl and stir until fully incorporated.

5. Arrange the vegetable sauce in a thin layer in the bottom of a 9 by 13-inch baking dish. Cover the sauce with a layer of lasagna noodles.

6. Put the noodles with half of the ricotta mixture on top, followed by half of the veggie sauce and a third of the mozzarella cheese..

7. Repeat layers, ending with a layer of noodles topped with the remaining mozzarella and all of the Parmesan cheese.

8. Cover with foil and bake for 25 minutes. Remove foil and bake for another 20 minutes, or until cheese is bubbly and golden.

9. Let stand for 10 minutes before slicing and serving.

Per serving: Calories: 450; Fat: 22g; Protein: 25g; Carbs: 40g; Sugar: 6g; Fiber: 5g

Difficulty rating: ★★★☆☆

70. Vegetarian Shepherd's Pie

Prep time: 25 minutes

Cook time: 30 minutes

Serves: 4

Ingredients:

- 2 tablespoons garlic-infused olive oil

- 1 medium carrot, diced

- 1 celery stalk, diced

- 1/2 cup diced bell pepper

- 1 cup cooked red lentils (use no more than ½ cup per serving to remain low-FODMAP)

- 2 cups low-FODMAP vegetable broth

- 1 teaspoon dried thyme

- 1 teaspoon dried rosemary

- Salt and pepper, to taste

- 2 pounds potatoes, peeled and cubed

- 1/4 cup lactose-free milk

- 2 tablespoons vegan butter

- 1/4 cup grated vegan cheese (optional)

Preparation instructions:

1. Preheat the oven to 375°F (190°C).

2. Heat 1 tablespoon of garlic-infused olive oil in a large pan over medium heat. Add carrot, celery, and bell pepper. Cook for 5-7 minutes until softened.

3. Stir in lentils, vegetable broth, thyme, rosemary, salt, and pepper. Bring to a boil, then reduce heat and simmer for 20-25 minutes, or until lentils are tender.

4. Meanwhile, place potatoes in a large pot and cover with water. Bring to a boil and cook until tender, about 15-20 minutes. Drain and return potatoes to the pot.

5. Add lactose-free milk, vegan butter, and mash until smooth. Season with salt and pepper to taste.

6. Spoon the lentil mixture into an ovenproof dish. On top, distribute the mashed potatoes. If used, scatter with vegan cheese.

7. Bake for 20-25 minutes, or until the top is golden and crispy.

8. Let cool for a few minutes before serving.

Per serving: Calories: 450; Fat: 14g; Protein: 18g; Carbs: 68g; Sugar: 8g; Fiber: 14g

Difficulty rating: ★★★☆☆

71. Vegan Lentil & Vegetable Curry

Prep time: 20 minutes

Cook time: 25 minutes

Serves: 4

Ingredients:

- 1 tablespoon olive oil

- 1 large carrot, peeled and diced

- 1 red bell pepper, diced

- 1 zucchini, diced

- 1¼ cups canned lentils, rinsed and drained (divided into ¼ cup per serving to remain low-FODMAP)

- 1 can (14 oz) diced tomatoes, no onion or garlic

- 1 can (14 oz / 400ml) unsweetened UHT coconut milk (use UHT type to stay within low-FODMAP limits at 100ml per serving)

- 2 tablespoons curry powder

- 1 teaspoon turmeric

- 1 teaspoon cumin

- 1/2 teaspoon salt

- 1/4 teaspoon black pepper

- 1/4 cup cilantro, chopped for garnish

- Cooked rice, for serving

Preparation instructions:

1. Heat the olive oil in a large skillet over medium heat. Add the carrot, red bell pepper, and zucchini. Cook for 5-7 minutes, or until the vegetables are slightly softened.

2. Stir in the canned lentils, diced tomatoes, coconut milk, curry powder, turmeric, cumin, salt, and black pepper. Bring the mixture to a simmer.

3. After lowering the heat to low, stew the vegetables for 15 to 20 minutes, stirring now and again, until they are soft and the flavors are combined.

4. Serve the curry over cooked rice and garnish with chopped cilantro.

Per serving: Calories: 345; Fat: 17g; Protein: 9g; Carbs: 39g; Sugar: 6g; Fiber: 7g

Difficulty rating: ★★★☆☆

Fish and Seafood

72. Grilled Mahi Mahi with Pineapple Salsa

Prep time: 20 minutes

Cook time: 10 minutes

Serves: 4

Ingredients:

- 4 Mahi Mahi fillets (about 6 ounces each)
- 2 tablespoons olive oil
- Salt and pepper, to taste
- 1 cup pineapple, diced
- 1/4 cup red bell pepper, diced
- 1/4 cup cucumber, diced
- 1/2 cup chopped green onions (green parts only)
- 1 jalapeño, seeded and finely chopped
- 2 tablespoons fresh cilantro, chopped
- Juice of 1 lime
- 1 maple syrup

Directions:

1. Preheat the grill to medium-high heat.

2. Brush the Mahi Mahi fillets with olive oil and season with salt and pepper.

3. Grill the fillets for about 4-5 minutes on each side, or until the fish flakes easily with a fork.

4. In a medium bowl, combine the pineapple, red bell pepper, cucumber, green onion, jalapeño, cilantro, lime juice, and maple syrup. Stir well to mix.

5. Season the salsa with salt and pepper to taste.

6. Serve the grilled Mahi Mahi topped with the pineapple salsa.

Per serving: Calories: 250; Fat: 9g; Protein: 23g; Carbs: 19g; Sugar: 14g; Fiber: 2g

Difficulty rating: ★★★☆☆

---

73. Baked Lemon Butter Tilapia

Prep time: 10 minutes

Cook time: 20 minutes

Serves: 4

Ingredients:

- 4 tilapia fillets (about 6 ounces each)
- 2 tablespoons olive oil
- 2 tablespoons unsalted butter, melted
- 1 lemon, juiced
- 1 teaspoon garlic-infused olive oil
- Salt and pepper, to taste
- 1 tablespoon fresh parsley, chopped
- Lemon slices, for garnish

Preparation instructions:

1. Set oven temperature to 400°F, or 200°C. A baking sheet can be lightly oiled with olive oil or lined with parchment paper.

2. Place the tilapia fillets on the prepared baking sheet.

3. In a small bowl, mix together the olive oil, melted butter, lemon juice, and garlic-infused olive oil. Season with salt and pepper to taste.

4. Pour the lemon butter mixture over the tilapia fillets, ensuring each fillet is well coated.

5. Bake for 15 to 20 minutes in a preheated oven, or until a fork can easily pierce the fish.

6. Remove from the oven and sprinkle with fresh parsley. Garnish with lemon slices before serving.

Per serving: Calories: 230; Fat: 15g; Protein: 23g; Carbs: 1g; Sugar: 0g; Fiber: 0g

Difficulty rating: ★☆☆☆☆

Allergen information: Gluten-free, Dairy-free option (substitute butter with additional olive oil).

---

74. Butter Shrimp Scampi

Prep time: 15 minutes

Cook time: 10 minutes

Serves: 4

Ingredients:

- 1 lb large shrimp, peeled and deveined
- 2 tablespoons garlic-infused olive oil
- 3 tablespoons unsalted butter
- 1/4 cup low-FODMAP chicken broth
- 1 tablespoon fresh lemon juice
- 1/2 teaspoon red pepper flakes (optional)
- Salt and pepper, to taste
- 2 tablespoons fresh parsley, finely chopped
- Lemon wedges, for serving

Preparation instructions:

1. Heat the garlic-infused olive oil and butter in a large skillet over medium heat until the butter is melted.

2. Add the shrimp to the skillet and season with salt and pepper. Cook for 1-2 minutes on one side until they start to turn pink.

3. Flip the shrimp and add the chicken broth, lemon juice, and red pepper flakes (if using). Cook for another 2-3 minutes, or until the shrimp are cooked through and the sauce has slightly thickened.

4. Remove from heat and stir in the chopped parsley.

5. Serve immediately with lemon wedges on the side.

Per serving: Calories: 230; Fat: 15g; Protein: 23g; Carbs: 1g; Sugar: 0g; Fiber: 0g

Difficulty rating: ★★☆☆☆

Prep time: 15 minutes

Cook time: 10 minutes

Serves: 4

Ingredients:

- 4 catfish fillets (about 6 ounces each)
- 2 tablespoons garlic-infused olive oil
- 1 tablespoon paprika
- 2 teaspoons dried thyme
- 1 teaspoon dried oregano
- 1/2 teaspoon cayenne pepper
- 1/2 teaspoon salt
- 1/4 teaspoon black pepper
- Lemon wedges, for serving

Preparation instructions:

1. In a small bowl, mix together paprika, dried thyme, dried oregano, cayenne pepper, salt, and black pepper to create the Cajun seasoning.

2. After giving the catfish fillets a quick rinse in cold water, blot dry using paper towels.

3. Rub each fillet evenly with garlic-infused olive oil, then coat generously with the Cajun seasoning mix.

4. Heat a large skillet over medium-high heat. Once hot, add the seasoned catfish fillets.

5. Cook for about 4-5 minutes on each side, or until the fish is opaque and flakes easily with a fork.

6. Serve hot, accompanied by lemon wedges.

Per serving: Calories: 280; Fat: 15g; Protein: 34g; Carbohydrates: 2g; Sugar: 0g; Fiber: 1g

Difficulty rating: ★★☆☆☆

Prep time: 15 minutes

Cook time: 15 minutes

Serves: 4

Ingredients:

- 4 salmon fillets (6 ounces each)
- 2 tablespoons garlic-infused olive oil
- 3 tablespoons pure maple syrup
- 2 tablespoons gluten-free soy sauce
- 1 tablespoon fresh lemon juice
- 1 teaspoon ground ginger
- Salt and pepper, to taste
- Fresh parsley, chopped (for garnish)
- Lemon slices (for serving)

Preparation instructions:

1. Preheat your oven to 375°F (190°C). Line a baking sheet with parchment paper.

2. In a small bowl, whisk together garlic-infused olive oil, maple syrup, gluten-free soy sauce, lemon juice, and ground ginger.

3. Put the salmon fillets onto the baking sheet that has been prepared. Use salt and pepper to season each fillet.

4. Evenly pour the maple syrup mixture over the salmon fillets.

5. Bake in the preheated oven for 12-15 minutes, or until salmon is opaque and flakes easily with a fork.

6. Remove from the oven and garnish with fresh parsley. Serve with lemon slices on the side.

Per serving: Calories: 295; Fat: 13g; Protein: 23g; Carbohydrates: 19g; Sugar: 17g; Fiber: 0g

Difficulty rating: ★★☆☆

Allergen information: Gluten-free.

---

77. Spicy Tuna Poke Bowl

Prep time: 20 minutes

Cook time: 0 minutes

Serves: 2

Ingredients:

- 8 oz sushi-grade tuna, diced

- 1/4 cup cucumber, diced

- 1/4 cup radishes, thinly sliced

- 2 tablespoons green onions (green parts only), thinly sliced

- 2 tablespoons gluten-free soy sauce or tamari

- 1 tablespoon sesame oil

- 1 teaspoon rice vinegar

- 1/2 teaspoon ginger, grated

- 1 teaspoon sesame seeds, plus extra for decoration

- Salt and pepper, to taste

- Cooked rice or quinoa, for serving (optional)

Directions:

1. Combine the chopped tuna, green onions, cucumber, and radishes in a big bowl.

2. To make the dressing, combine the sesame oil, rice vinegar, grated ginger, and gluten-free soy sauce or tamari in a small bowl.

3. Drizzle the tuna mixture with the dressing, then gently toss to evenly coat all the ingredients.

4. Add pepper and salt to taste, and then top with sesame seeds.

5. Serve the spicy tuna poke over a bed of cooked rice or quinoa if desired, and garnish with additional sesame seeds.

Per serving: Calories: 340; Fat: 20g; Protein: 33g; Carbs: 10g; Sugar: 2g; Fiber: 3g

Difficulty rating: ★☆☆☆

Allergen information: Gluten-free, Dairy-free, Nut-free

78. *Tropical Coconut Shrimp Delight*

Prep time: 20 minutes

Cook time: 10 minutes

Serves: 4

Ingredients:

- 24 large shrimp, peeled and deveined

- 1/2 cup unsweetened shredded coconut

- 1/2 cup gluten-free breadcrumbs

- 2 large eggs, beaten

- 1/4 cup cornstarch

- Salt and pepper, to taste

- 1/4 cup garlic-infused olive oil, for frying

For the Pineapple Dipping Sauce:

- 1 cup fresh pineapple, peeled and chopped

- 1 tablespoon lime juice

- 1 teaspoon rice vinegar

- 1/4 teaspoon red pepper flakes

- Salt, to taste

Directions:

1. Pat the shrimp dry with paper towels to prepare them. Add pepper and salt for seasoning.

2. Set up three shallow bowls for the breading process: one with cornstarch, one with beaten eggs, and one with a mixture of shredded coconut and gluten-free breadcrumbs.

3. Coat each shrimp first in cornstarch, shaking off the excess, then dip into the beaten eggs, and finally coat with the coconut-breadcrumb mixture.

4. In a large skillet, heat the garlic-infused oil over medium heat. Fry the shrimp in batches for 2 to 3 minutes on each side, or until they are crispy and golden brown. Transfer to a plate covered with paper towels to drain.

5. For the pineapple dipping sauce, blend the pineapple, lime juice, rice vinegar, red pepper flakes, and salt in a blender until smooth.

6. Serve the crispy coconut shrimp with the pineapple dipping sauce on the side.

Per serving: Calories: 350; Fat: 18g; Protein: 15g; Carbs: 30g; Sugar: 8g; Fiber: 2g

Difficulty rating: ★★☆☆☆

---

79. *Pan-Seared Scallops with Lemon Herb Sauce*

Prep time: 15 minutes

Cook time: 10 minutes

Serves: 4

Ingredients:

- 12 large sea scallops, patted dry

- 2 tablespoons garlic-infused olive oil

- Salt and pepper, to taste

- 1 tablespoon unsalted butter

- 1/4 cup fresh lemon juice

- 1 tablespoon fresh parsley, chopped

- 1 teaspoon fresh thyme leaves

- Lemon wedges, for serving

Preparation instructions:

1. Heat the garlic-infused olive oil in a large skillet over medium-high heat.

2. Season the scallops with salt and pepper. Once the skillet is hot, add the scallops, making sure not to overcrowd the pan. Cook for about 2-3 minutes on one side until a golden crust forms.

3. Flip the scallops and add the butter, lemon juice, parsley, and thyme to the skillet. Cook for another 2-3 minutes, spooning the butter and lemon sauce over the scallops as they cook.

4. Remove the scallops from the skillet and arrange them on a serving platter. Pour the lemon herb sauce from the skillet over the scallops.

5. Serve immediately with lemon wedges on the side.

Per serving: Calories: 200; Fat: 12g; Protein: 14g; Carbs: 5g; Sugar: 0g; Fiber: 0g

Difficulty rating: ★★☆☆☆

Allergen information: Gluten-free, Dairy-free option (omit butter or use a dairy-free alternative).

---

80. Baked Halibut with Tomato Basil Sauce

Prep time: 20 minutes

Cook time: 25 minutes

Serves: 4

Ingredients:

- 4 halibut fillets (about 6 ounces each)
- Salt and pepper, to taste
- 2 tablespoons garlic-infused olive oil
- 1 can (14 oz) diced tomatoes, drained
- 1/4 cup fresh basil, chopped
- 1 tablespoon balsamic vinegar
- 1 teaspoon dried oregano
- 1/4 teaspoon red pepper flakes (optional)

Preparation instructions:

1. Preheat the oven to 375°F (190°C). Season the halibut fillets with salt and pepper on both sides.

2. Heat 1 tablespoon of garlic-infused olive oil in a large ovenproof skillet over medium-high heat. Add the halibut fillets and sear for about 2 minutes on each side, or until golden brown. Remove the fillets from the skillet and set aside.

3. Add the last tablespoon of garlic-infused oil to the same skillet.

4. To the skillet, add the red pepper flakes (if using), chopped basil, balsamic vinegar, dry oregano, and diced tomatoes that have been drained. After combining, cook for two to three minutes.

5. Return the halibut fillets to the skillet, spooning the tomato basil sauce over them.

6. Transfer the skillet to the preheated oven and bake for 15-20 minutes, or until the halibut is cooked through and flakes easily with a fork.

7. Serve the baked halibut with additional sauce spooned over the top.

Per serving: Calories: 280; Fat: 10g; Protein: 35g; Carbs: 8g; Sugar: 4g; Fiber: 2g

Difficulty rating: ★★☆☆☆

---

81. Grilled Swordfish with Chimichurri

Prep time: 20 minutes

Cook time: 12 minutes

Serves: 4

Ingredients:

- 4 swordfish steaks (about 6 ounces each)
- 2 tablespoons olive oil
- Salt and pepper, to taste
- 1 cup fresh parsley, finely chopped
- 1/4 cup garlic-infused olive oil
- 2 tablespoons red wine vinegar
- 1 teaspoon red chili flakes
- 1 teaspoon dried oregano
- Salt and pepper, to taste

Preparation instructions:

1. Preheat the grill to medium-high. Brush swordfish steaks with olive oil and season with salt and pepper.

2. Grill for 5–6 minutes per side, until the fish flakes easily with a fork.

3. Meanwhile, mix parsley, garlic-infused olive oil, red wine vinegar, chili flakes, oregano, salt, and pepper to make the chimichurri.

4. Let the swordfish rest for a few minutes, then serve with the chimichurri sauce on top or on the side.

Per serving: Calories: 380; Fat: 28g; Protein: 27g; Carbohydrates: 2g; Sugar: 0g; Fiber: 0.5g

Difficulty rating: ★★☆☆☆

82. Shrimp and Cucumber Salad

Prep time: 15 minutes

Cook time: 0 minutes

Serves: 4

Ingredients:

- 1 lb cooked shrimp, peeled and deveined
- 3/4 cup cucumber, diced
- 1/4 cup red bell pepper, diced
- 2 tablespoons fresh lime juice
- 1 tablespoon garlic-infused olive oil
- 1/4 teaspoon salt
- 1/4 teaspoon black pepper
- 2 tablespoons fresh cilantro, chopped
- Mixed greens for serving

Preparation instructions:

1. In a large mixing bowl, combine the cooked shrimp, diced cucumber, and red bell pepper.

2. In a small bowl, whisk together the fresh lime juice, garlic-infused olive oil, salt, and black pepper.

3. Pour the dressing over the shrimp mixture. Gently toss to coat all the ingredients evenly.

4. Fold in the chopped fresh cilantro.

5. Serve the salad over a bed of mixed greens.

Per serving: Calories: 240; Fat: 12g; Protein: 25g; Carbohydrates: 8g; Sugar: 3g; Fiber: 3g

Prep time: 15 minutes

Cook time: 20 minutes

Serves: 4

Ingredients:

- 4 cod fillets (about 6 ounces each)

- 2 tablespoons garlic-infused olive oil

- 1/4 teaspoon salt

- 1/4 teaspoon black pepper

- 1 tablespoon fresh dill, chopped, plus extra for garnish

- 1 lemon, thinly sliced

Preparation instructions:

1. Preheat the oven to 400°F (200°C). Line a baking sheet with parchment paper.

2. Place the cod fillets on the prepared baking sheet. Brush each fillet evenly with garlic-infused olive oil.

3. Season the fillets with salt and black pepper.

4. Arrange lemon slices on and around the cod fillets.

5. Bake in the preheated oven for 18-20 minutes, or until the fish flakes easily with a fork.

6. Garnish with additional fresh dill before serving.

Per serving: Calories: 190; Fat: 7g; Protein: 30g; Carbs: 2g; Sugar: 0g; Fiber: 0g

Difficulty rating: ★☆☆☆☆

Poultry and Meat

84. Lemon Herb Chicken Thighs

Prep time: 20 minutes

Cook time: 25 minutes

Serves: 4

Ingredients:

- 4 chicken thighs, bone-in and skin-on
- 2 tablespoons garlic-infused oil
- 1 tablespoon fresh lemon juice
- 1 tablespoon fresh rosemary, chopped
- 1 tablespoon fresh thyme, chopped
- Salt and pepper, to taste
- Lemon slices, for garnish
- Additional fresh herbs, for garnish

Preparation instructions:

1. Preheat the oven to 375°F (190°C).

2. In a small bowl, whisk together garlic-infused oil, lemon juice, rosemary, thyme, salt, and pepper.

3. The chicken thighs ought to be put in a baking dish. Make sure the chicken thighs are thoroughly covered by brushing both sides with the oil and herb mixture.

4. Arrange lemon slices around the chicken in the baking dish.

5. Bake in the preheated oven for 25 minutes, or until the chicken is cooked through and the skin is golden and crispy.

6. Remove from the oven and let rest for 5 minutes before serving. Garnish with additional fresh herbs.

Per serving: Calories: 310; Fat: 22g; Protein: 24g; Carbs: 1g; Sugar: 0g; Fiber: 0g

Difficulty rating: ★☆☆☆☆

Allergen information: Gluten-free, Dairy-free.

85. Rosemary Pork Chops

Prep time: 15 minutes

Cook time: 25 minutes

Serves: 4

Ingredients:

- 4 pork chops, about 1 inch thick
- 2 tablespoons garlic-infused olive oil
- 2 tablespoons fresh rosemary, chopped
- Salt and pepper, to taste

Preparation instructions:

1. Preheat your oven to 375°F (190°C).

2. Rub each pork chop with garlic-infused olive oil, then season both sides with salt and pepper.

3. Sprinkle the chopped rosemary evenly over each pork chop, pressing gently to adhere the herbs to the meat.

4. Heat a large oven-proof skillet over medium-high heat. Once hot, add the pork chops and sear for about 3-4 minutes on each side, or until they develop a golden crust.

5. After placing the skillet in the oven, bake it for 15 to 20 minutes, or until the internal temperature of the pork chops reaches 145°F (63°C).

6. Prior to serving, allow the pork chops to rest for five minutes so that the liquids can redistribute.

Per serving: Calories: 290; Fat: 16g; Protein: 30g; Carbs: 1g; Sugar: 0g; Fiber: 0g

Difficulty rating: ★★☆☆☆

Allergen information: Gluten-free, Dairy-free.

86. Maple Mustard Chicken Breasts

Prep time: 15 minutes

Cook time: 25 minutes

Serves: 4

Ingredients:

- 4 boneless, skinless chicken breasts
- Salt and pepper, to taste
- 2 tablespoons olive oil
- 1/4 cup pure maple syrup
- 1/4 cup Dijon mustard
- 1 tablespoon apple cider vinegar
- 1 teaspoon dried thyme
- 1/2 teaspoon paprika

Preparation instructions:

1. Preheat the oven to 375°F (190°C). Season the chicken breasts with salt and pepper on both sides.

2. In a large ovenproof skillet, heat the olive oil over medium-high heat. Add the chicken breasts and sear for 3–4 minutes on each side, or until golden brown. After taking the chicken out of the skillet, set it aside.

3. In the same skillet, reduce the heat to low and add the maple syrup, Dijon mustard, apple cider vinegar, dried thyme, and paprika. Stir to combine and cook for 1-2 minutes, until the sauce is smooth and slightly thickened.

4. Return the chicken breasts to the skillet, spooning the sauce over them to coat evenly.

5. After transferring the skillet to the preheated oven, bake it for 20 minutes, or until the internal temperature of the chicken reaches 165°F (74°C) and it is thoroughly cooked.

6. Serve the chicken breasts with extra sauce from the skillet drizzled on top.

Per serving: Calories: 320; Fat: 10g; Protein: 27g; Carbs: 30g; Sugar: 27g; Fiber: 0g

Difficulty rating: ★★☆☆☆

Allergen information: Gluten-free.

---

87. Spicy Beef Tacos

Prep time: 20 minutes

Cook time: 10 minutes

Serves: 4

Ingredients:

- 1 lb lean ground beef

- 1 tablespoon garlic-infused olive oil

- 1 teaspoon cumin

- 1 teaspoon smoked paprika

- 1/2 teaspoon chili powder

- 1/4 teaspoon salt

- 1/4 teaspoon black pepper

- 8 gluten-free corn tortillas

- 1/2 cup diced tomatoes (ensure no onion or garlic for low-FODMAP)

- 1/2 cup shredded lettuce

- 1/2 cup grated cheddar cheese (lactose-free if necessary)

- 1/4 cup chopped fresh cilantro

- Lime wedges, for serving

Directions:

1. In a large skillet, heat the garlic-infused olive oil over medium heat. Add the ground beef and simmer, breaking it up with a spoon, for 5 to 7 minutes, or until browned.

2. Stir in cumin, smoked paprika, chili powder, salt, and pepper. Cook for an additional 2-3 minutes, until the beef is well seasoned.

3. Warm the corn tortillas according to package instructions.

4. To assemble the tacos, divide the cooked beef among the tortillas.

5. Top each taco with diced tomatoes, shredded lettuce, grated cheddar cheese, and chopped cilantro.

6. Serve with lime wedges on the side.

Per serving: Calories: 350; Fat: 15g; Protein: 25g; Carbs: 25g; Sugar: 2g; Fiber: 3g

Difficulty rating: ★☆☆☆☆

Allergen information: Gluten-free, Dairy-free option (omit cheese or use dairy-free cheese).

---

88. Herb-Crusted Lamb Chops

Prep time: 15 minutes

Cook time: 15 minutes

Serves: 4

Ingredients:

- 8 lamb chops
- 2 tablespoons garlic-infused olive oil
- 1/4 cup fresh rosemary, finely chopped
- 1/4 cup fresh thyme, finely chopped
- Salt and pepper, to taste
- 1 tablespoon Dijon mustard
- 1/2 cup gluten-free breadcrumbs

Preparation instructions:

1. Preheat the grill to medium-high heat.

2. Rub each lamb chop with garlic-infused olive oil, then season both sides with salt and pepper.

3. In a small bowl, mix together the rosemary, thyme, and Dijon mustard. Spread this mixture over one side of each lamb chop.

4. Press the gluten-free breadcrumbs onto the mustard-herb mixture to coat.

5. Place the lamb chops on the grill, breadcrumb side up, and cook for about 7-8 minutes. Flip the chops and grill for another 7-8 minutes for medium-rare, or until they reach your desired level of doneness.

6. Let the lamb chops rest for a few minutes before serving.

Per serving: Calories: 320; Fat: 18g; Protein: 34g; Carbs: 8g; Sugar: 1g; Fiber: 1g

Difficulty rating: ★★☆☆☆

Allergen information: Gluten-free, Dairy-free.

---

89. Teriyaki Chicken Skewers

Prep time: 20 minutes

Cook time: 10 minutes

Serves: 4

Ingredients:

- 1 lb chicken breast, cut into 1-inch pieces
- 1/4 cup low-sodium soy sauce (ensure gluten-free for a low-FODMAP diet)
- 2 tablespoons maple syrup
- 1 tablespoon rice vinegar
- 1 tablespoon garlic-infused olive oil
- 1 teaspoon ginger, grated
- Salt and pepper, to taste
- 1 tablespoon sesame oil
- 1 red bell pepper, cut into 1-inch pieces
- 1 green bell pepper, cut into 1-inch pieces
- 8 skewers (if wooden, soak in water for at least 30 minutes prior to use)

Preparation instructions:

1. In a bowl, whisk together soy sauce, maple syrup, rice vinegar, garlic-infused olive oil, grated ginger, salt, and pepper to create the marinade.

2. Make sure the chicken pieces are well covered after adding them to the marinade. If you want a deeper taste, cover and chill for up to 4 hours, but at least 30 minutes.

3. Set the grill's temperature to medium-high. Onto the skewers, alternately thread the marinated chicken and bell pepper pieces.

4. Brush the grill with sesame oil to prevent sticking. Grill the skewers for 5 minutes on each side, or until the chicken is cooked through and slightly charred.

5. Serve hot.

Per serving: Calories: 250; Fat: 9g; Protein: 26g; Carbs: 15g; Sugar: 10g; Fiber: 1g

Difficulty rating: ★★☆☆☆

---

90. Balsamic Glazed Pork Tenderloin

Prep time: 15 minutes

Cook time: 25 minutes

Serves: 4

Ingredients:

- 1 (1.5-pound) pork tenderloin

- 1/4 cup balsamic vinegar

- 2 tablespoons garlic-infused olive oil

- 2 tablespoons Dijon mustard

- 2 tablespoons maple syrup

- 1 teaspoon dried thyme

- 1/2 teaspoon salt

- 1/4 teaspoon black pepper

Directions:

1. Preheat the oven to 375°F (190°C).

2. In a small bowl, whisk together balsamic vinegar, garlic-infused olive oil, Dijon mustard, maple syrup, dried thyme, salt and black pepper to create the glaze.

3. Place the pork tenderloin in a baking dish. Brush the glaze generously over the tenderloin, ensuring it is well coated.

4. Roast for 25 minutes in a preheated oven, or until the pork achieves an internal temperature of 145°F (63°C).

5. Remove from the oven and let the pork tenderloin rest for 5 minutes before slicing.

6. Slice the pork tenderloin and serve with additional glaze drizzled on top if desired.

Per serving: Calories: 280; Fat: 10g; Protein: 35g; Carbs: 12g; Sugar: 10g; Fiber: 0g

Difficulty rating: ★★☆☆☆

Allergen information: Gluten-free, Dairy-free.

91. Cajun Spiced Chicken Wings

Prep time: 15 minutes

Cook time: 25 minutes

Serves: 4

Ingredients:

- 2 lbs chicken wings, separated into drumettes and flats
- 2 tablespoons olive oil
- 1 tablespoon smoked paprika
- 2 teaspoons dried thyme
- 2 teaspoons dried oregano
- 1 teaspoon cayenne pepper (adjust to taste)
- 1 teaspoon salt
- 1/2 teaspoon black pepper
- 1/4 cup fresh parsley, finely chopped, for garnish

Directions:

1. Preheat the oven to 425°F (220°C). Line a baking sheet with parchment paper or a silicone baking mat.

2. In a large bowl, toss the chicken wings with olive oil, smoked paprika, dried thyme, dried oregano, cayenne pepper, salt, and black pepper until evenly coated.

3. Arrange the wings in a single layer on the prepared baking sheet.

4 Bake the wings for 25 minutes, or until they are cooked through and crispy, in a preheated oven. To guarantee even crispiness, turn the wings halfway through the cooking process.

5. Remove from the oven and let cool slightly. Garnish with fresh parsley before serving.

Per serving: Calories: 310; Fat: 22g; Protein: 24g; Carbs: 2g; Sugar: 0g; Fiber: 1g

Difficulty rating: ★☆☆☆☆

---

92. Rosemary Roast Beef

Prep time: 20 minutes

Cook time: 60 minutes

Serves: 4

Ingredients:

- 2 lbs beef roast
- 2 tablespoons garlic-infused olive oil
- 1 tablespoon fresh rosemary, chopped
- 1 teaspoon salt
- 1/2 teaspoon black pepper
- 1/4 cup low-FODMAP beef broth
- 2 tablespoons balsamic vinegar
- 1 tablespoon Dijon mustard
- 1 teaspoon dried thyme

Preparation instructions:

1. Preheat your oven to 375°F (190°C).

2. Rub the beef roast evenly with garlic-infused olive oil, then season with chopped rosemary, salt, and black pepper.

3. The roast should be put in a roasting pan. Combine the dried thyme, balsamic vinegar, Dijon mustard, and low-FODMAP beef broth in a small bowl. Cover the roast with this mixture.

4. Roast in the preheated oven for about 60 minutes, or until the internal temperature reaches 145°F (63°C) for medium-rare.

5. Before slicing, take the roast out of the oven and give it ten minutes to rest. This keeps the meat moist and tasty by allowing the liquids to re-distribute throughout the flesh.

6. Slice the roast beef and serve with the pan juices drizzled on top.

Per serving: Calories: 480; Fat: 34g; Protein: 38g; Carbs: 2g; Sugar: 1g; Fiber: 0g

Difficulty rating: ★★☆☆☆

Allergen information: Gluten-free, Dairy-free.

---

93. BBQ Pulled Pork

Prep time: 20 minutes

Cook time: 8 hours (slow cooker on low) | 4 hours (slow cooker on high)

Serves: 6

Ingredients:

- 2 lbs pork shoulder

- 2 tablespoons garlic-infused olive oil

- 1 cup low-FODMAP BBQ sauce

- 1/2 cup water

- 1 tablespoon brown sugar

- 1 tablespoon smoked paprika

- 1 teaspoon salt

- 1/2 teaspoon black pepper

- 1/4 teaspoon cayenne pepper (optional)

- 6 gluten-free hamburger buns

Directions:

1. Rub the pork shoulder all over with the garlic-infused olive oil.

2. In a small bowl, mix together the brown sugar, smoked paprika, salt, black pepper, and cayenne pepper. Rub this mixture onto the pork shoulder.

3. Place the seasoned pork shoulder in the slow cooker. Pour the water and low-FODMAP BBQ sauce over the pork.

4. Cook the pork covered for 8 hours on low or 4 hours on high, or until it is very soft and readily shreds with a fork.

5. Remove the pork from the slow cooker and shred it using two forks. Return the shredded pork to the slow cooker and stir it into the sauce.

6. Serve the BBQ pulled pork on gluten-free hamburger buns.

Per serving: Calories: 510; Fat: 22g; Protein: 35g; Carbs: 45g; Sugar: 15g; Fiber: 2g

Difficulty rating: ★☆☆☆☆

Allergen information: Gluten-free, Dairy-free.

94. Stuffed Chicken Breasts with Spinach and Feta

Prep time: 20 minutes

Cook time: 30 minutes

Serves: 4

Ingredients:

- 4 boneless, skinless chicken breasts

- 1 cup baby spinach, chopped

- 1/2 cup feta cheese, crumbled

- 2 tablespoons olive oil

- Salt and pepper, to taste

- 1/2 teaspoon dried oregano

- Toothpicks or kitchen twine

Directions:

1. Preheat your oven to 375°F (190°C).

2. Place the breasts of chicken flat on a chopping board. Slice each breast horizontally to form a pocket with a sharp knife, taking care not to cut all the way through.

3. Combine the crumbled feta cheese and chopped spinach in a bowl. Place the spinach and feta mixture into each chicken breast and fasten the openings with kitchen twine or toothpicks.

4. Season the outside of the chicken breasts with salt, pepper, and dried oregano.

5. Heat olive oil in a large, oven-safe skillet over medium-high heat. Add the stuffed chicken breasts to the skillet and sear for about 3 minutes on each side, or until golden brown.

6. After transferring the skillet to the oven, warm it and bake for 20 to 25 minutes, or until the chicken is thoroughly cooked and the middle is no longer pink..

7. Remove from the oven and let the chicken rest for a few minutes before removing the toothpicks or twine. Serve warm.

Per serving: Calories: 290; Fat: 15g; Protein: 34g; Carbs: 2g; Sugar: 1g; Fiber: 0.5g

Difficulty rating: ★★☆☆☆

Allergen information: Gluten-free, Nut-free.

95. Beef and Mushroom Stroganoff

Prep time: 20 minutes

Cook time: 25 minutes

Serves: 4

Ingredients:

- 1 lb beef sirloin, thinly sliced

- 2 tablespoons garlic-infused olive oil

- 1 cup beef broth (low-FODMAP)

- 1 cup lactose-free sour cream

- 1½ cups oyster mushrooms, sliced

- 1 tablespoon Worcestershire sauce (ensure gluten-free)

- 1 teaspoon Dijon mustard

- 1/4 teaspoon salt

- 1/4 teaspoon black pepper

- 2 tablespoons fresh parsley, chopped

- Cooked gluten-free pasta or rice, for serving

Preparation instructions:

1. In a large skillet over medium-high heat, heat 1 tablespoon of garlic-infused oil. After adding the steak pieces, sauté them for three to five minutes, or until they are browned all over. Take out and reserve the steak from the skillet..

2. Place the sliced oyster mushrooms and the last tablespoon of garlic-infused oil in the same skillet. Simmer for 5 to 7 minutes, or until the mushrooms are tender and caramelized.

3. Set the temperature to medium. Put the steak back in the skillet along with the Worcestershire sauce, Dijon mustard, and beef broth. Mix thoroughly to blend.

4. Slowly stir in the lactose-free sour cream until the mixture is well combined and heated through, but do not boil. Season with salt and pepper.

5. Garnish with fresh parsley before serving.

6. Serve the beef and mushroom stroganoff over cooked gluten-free pasta or rice.

Per serving: Calories: 315; Fat: 17g; Protein: 25g: Carbs: 11g; Sugar: 2g; Fiber: 1g

Difficulty rating: ★★☆☆☆

Allergen information: Gluten-free, Lactose-free.

Soups and Salads

96. Roasted Red Pepper Soup

Prep time: 15 minutes

Cook time: 25 minutes

Serves: 4

Ingredients:

- 4 large red bell peppers, halved and seeds removed
- 1 tablespoon garlic-infused olive oil
- 3 cups low-FODMAP vegetable broth
- 1 teaspoon smoked paprika
- 1/2 teaspoon ground cumin
- Salt and pepper, to taste
- 1/4 cup lactose-free cream, for serving
- Fresh parsley, chopped, for garnish

Directions:

1. Preheat your oven to 425°F (220°C). Place the red bell peppers on a baking sheet, cut side down, and brush with garlic-infused olive oil.

2. Roast the peppers in the preheated oven for 20 minutes, or until the skins are charred and blistered. Remove from the oven and allow to cool slightly. Peel off the skins and discard them.

3. In a blender, puree the roasted peppers with low-FODMAP vegetable broth, smoked paprika, and ground cumin until smooth.

4. Transfer the pureed mixture to a saucepan and heat over medium heat. Season with salt and pepper to taste. Cook for 5 minutes, stirring occasionally.

5. Serve the soup hot, drizzled with lactose-free cream and garnished with fresh parsley.

Per serving: Calories: 120; Fat: 7g; Protein: 2g; Carbs: 12g; Sugar: 6g; Fiber: 3g

Difficulty rating: ★☆☆☆

Allergen information: Gluten-free, Dairy-free option (omit lactose-free cream).

---

97. Lemon Chicken Rice Soup

Prep time: 20 minutes

Cook time: 30 minutes

Serves: 4

Ingredients:

- 1 cup cooked white rice (or jasmine rice)
- 2 tablespoons garlic-infused olive oil
- 1 lb chicken breast, cut into bite-sized pieces
- 6 cups low-FODMAP chicken broth
- 1 cup carrots, diced
- 1 cup zucchini, diced
- 1 tablespoon lemon juice
- 1 teaspoon dried thyme
- 1 teaspoon dried oregano
- Salt and pepper, to taste
- 2 tablespoons fresh parsley, chopped
- Lemon slices, for garnish

Preparation instructions:

1. Cook the rice separately and set aside.

2. In a large pot, heat garlic-infused olive oil over medium heat. Add chicken pieces and sauté until golden and cooked through (about 5–7 minutes). Remove chicken and set aside.

3. In the same pot, sauté carrots for 5 minutes. Add zucchini and cook for another 3 minutes.

4. Pour in the low-FODMAP chicken broth and bring to a simmer. Stir in lemon juice, thyme, oregano, salt, and pepper. Simmer for 10 minutes to allow flavors to meld.

5. Return chicken to the pot, then stir in the cooked white rice and warm through.

6. Garnish with fresh parsley and lemon slices. Serve hot.

Per serving: Calories: 335; Fat: 8g; Protein: 28g; Carbs: 36g; Sugar: 3g; Fiber: 2g

Difficulty rating: ★★☆☆☆

Allergen information: Gluten-free (ensure orzo is gluten-free), Dairy-free.

---

98. Thai Coconut Shrimp Soup

Prep time: 20 minutes

Cook time: 25 minutes

Serves: 4

Ingredients:

- 1 lb large shrimp, peeled and deveined
- 1 tablespoon garlic-infused olive oil
- 1 can (14 oz) light coconut milk
- 1 cup low-FODMAP vegetable broth
- 1 tablespoon ginger, grated
- 1 tablespoon lime juice
- 1 red bell pepper, sliced into thin strips
- 1 cup bamboo shoots, drained
- 1 tablespoon low-FODMAP green curry paste
- 1 teaspoon brown sugar
- 1/2 teaspoon salt
- 1/4 cup fresh cilantro, chopped
- 1/4 cup green onion tops, sliced

Directions:

1. Heat the garlic-infused olive oil in a large pot over medium heat. Add the shrimp and cook until they turn pink, about 2-3 minutes per side. Remove the shrimp from the pot and set aside.

2. In the same pot, add the coconut milk, low-FODMAP vegetable broth, grated ginger, and lime juice. Stir well to combine.

3. Add the sliced red bell pepper, bamboo shoots, and green curry paste to the pot. Stir in the brown sugar and salt. Bring the mixture to a simmer and cook for 10 minutes, stirring occasionally.

4. Return the cooked shrimp to the pot and heat through for about 2 minutes.

5. Garnish the soup with sliced green onion tops and chopped cilantro.

Per serving: Calories: 295; Fat: 18g; Protein: 25g; Carbs: 9g; Sugar: 4g; Fiber: 1g

Difficulty rating: ★★☆☆☆

Allergen information: Gluten-free, Dairy-free.

---

99. Butternut Squash and Sage Soup

Prep time: 15 minutes

Cook time: 30 minutes

Serves: 4

Ingredients:

- 1 large butternut squash, peeled, seeded, and cubed

- 2 tablespoons garlic-infused olive oil

- 4 cups low-FODMAP vegetable broth

- 1 tablespoon fresh sage, chopped

- Salt and pepper, to taste

- 1/4 cup lactose-free cream (optional, for serving)

- Fresh sage leaves, for garnish

Preparation instructions:

1. In a large pot, warm the garlic-infused oil over medium heat. When the butternut squash is slightly softened, add the cubed squash and simmer, stirring periodically, for about five minutes..

2. Add the chopped sage to the pot and cook for an additional minute, until fragrant.

3. Pour in the low-FODMAP vegetable broth and bring the mixture to a boil. Once boiling, reduce the heat to low, cover, and simmer for about 20 minutes, or until the butternut squash is tender.

4. Puree the soup with an immersion blender until it's smooth. Alternatively, move the soup into a blender and purée it in batches after careful handling. If blending the soup, put it back in the pot.

5. Season the soup with salt and pepper to taste. If desired, stir in lactose-free cream for a creamier texture.

6. Serve the soup hot, garnished with fresh sage leaves.

Per serving: Calories: 180; Fat: 7g; Protein: 2g; Carbs: 29g; Sugar: 5g; Fiber: 5g

Difficulty rating: ★☆☆☆☆

Allergen information: Gluten-free, Dairy-free (without optional cream), Nut-free.

100. Kale and Quinoa Salad

Prep time: 15 minutes

Cook time: 0 minutes

Serves: 4

Ingredients:

- 1 cup quinoa, cooked and cooled

- 2 cups kale, stems removed and leaves finely chopped

- 1/2 cup cucumber, diced

- 1/2 cup cherry tomatoes, halved

- 1/2 cup green onions (green parts only), finely chopped

- 1/4 cup feta cheese, crumbled

- 1/4 cup almonds, sliced

- 2 tablespoons olive oil

- 2 tablespoons lemon juice

- 1 teaspoon Dijon mustard

- Salt and pepper, to taste

Directions:

1. Cooked quinoa, kale, cucumber, cherry tomatoes, green onion, feta cheese, and sliced almonds should all be combined in a big mixing bowl.

2. In a small bowl, whisk together the olive oil, lemon juice, Dijon mustard, salt, and pepper to create the dressing.

3. Pour the dressing over the salad and toss well to ensure everything is evenly coated.

4. Adjust the seasoning with additional salt and pepper if needed.

5. Serve immediately or chill in the refrigerator for 30 minutes before serving to allow the flavors to meld.

Per serving: Calories: 280; Fat: 15g; Protein: 9g; Carbs: 30g; Sugar: 3g; Fiber: 5g

Difficulty rating: ★☆☆☆☆

Allergen information: Gluten-free, Nut-free option (omit almonds), Dairy-free option (omit feta cheese).

101. Arugula and Strawberry Salad

Prep time: 15 minutes

Cook time: 0 minutes

Serves: 4

Ingredients:

- 4 cups arugula, washed and dried

- 1/2 cup strawberries, hulled and thinly sliced

- 1/4 cup walnuts, toasted and chopped

- 1/4 cup crumbled feta cheese (lactose-free if necessary)

- 2 tablespoons olive oil

- 1 tablespoon balsamic vinegar

- 1 teaspoon Dijon mustard

- Salt and pepper, to taste

Directions:

1. In a large salad bowl, combine the arugula, sliced strawberries, toasted walnuts, and crumbled feta cheese.

2. In a small bowl, whisk together the olive oil, balsamic vinegar, Dijon mustard, salt, and pepper to create the dressing.

3. Pour the dressing over the salad and gently toss to combine.

4. Serve immediately, divided among four plates.

Per serving: Calories: 170; Fat: 14g; Protein: 4g; Carbs: 9g; Sugar: 4g; Fiber: 2g

Difficulty rating: ★☆☆☆☆

Allergen information: Gluten-free, Nut-free, Dairy-free option (omit feta or use dairy-free cheese).

102. Cantaloupe and Feta Salad

Prep time: 15 minutes

Cook time: 0 minutes

Serves: 4

Ingredients:

- 4 cups cubed cantaloupe

- 1 cup crumbled feta cheese (lactose-free or regular, max 40g per serving)

- 1/2 cup fresh mint leaves, chopped

- 2 tablespoons olive oil

- 1 tablespoon balsamic vinegar

- Salt and pepper, to taste

- 1/4 cup sliced almonds, toasted (for garnish)

Directions:

1. In a large bowl, combine the cubed cantaloupe, crumbled feta cheese, and chopped mint leaves.

2. Combine the balsamic vinegar and olive oil in a small basin. To taste, add salt and pepper for seasoning.

3. Pour the dressing over the mixture of cantaloupe and toss to blend lightly.

4. Serve the salad garnished with toasted sliced almonds.

Per serving: Calories: 180; Fat: 12g; Protein: 6g; Carbs: 14g; Sugar: 10g; Fiber: 1g

Difficulty rating: ★☆☆☆☆

Allergen information: Gluten-free, Nut-free option (omit almonds); Dairy-free option (use dairy-free feta).

103. Asian Cabbage Salad

Prep time: 15 minutes

Cook time: 0 minutes

Serves: 4

Ingredients:

- 4 cups shredded Napa cabbage

- 1 cup shredded carrots

- 1/2 cup thinly sliced red bell pepper

- 1/4 cup chopped green onions (green parts only)

- 1/4 cup chopped fresh cilantro

- 2 tablespoons sesame seeds

- 1/4 cup rice vinegar

- 2 tablespoons garlic-infused olive oil

- 1 tablespoon soy sauce (ensure gluten-free for a low-FODMAP diet)

- 1 tablespoon maple syrup

- 1 teaspoon grated ginger

- Salt and pepper, to taste

Preparation instructions:

1. In a large bowl, combine the shredded Napa cabbage, shredded carrots, thinly sliced red bell pepper, chopped green onions, and chopped fresh cilantro.

2. In a small bowl, whisk together the rice vinegar, garlic-infused olive oil, soy sauce, maple syrup, and grated ginger to create the dressing.

3. Pour the dressing over the cabbage mixture and toss well to coat all the ingredients evenly.

4. Season with salt and pepper to taste.

5. Sprinkle sesame seeds over the salad just before serving.

Per serving: Calories: 150; Fat: 7g; Protein: 3g; Carbs: 20g; Sugar: 10g; Fiber: 4g

Difficulty rating: ★☆☆☆☆

Allergen information: Gluten-free, Nut-free, Dairy-free.

---

104. Rustic Beet and Cheese Salad

Prep time: 20 minutes

Cook time: 0 minutes

Serves: 4

Ingredients:

- 4 medium beets, roasted, peeled, and sliced

- 4 cups mixed salad greens

- 1/2 cup walnuts, toasted and chopped

- 1/2 cup goat cheese, crumbled

- 2 tablespoons balsamic vinegar

- 4 tablespoons olive oil

- Salt and pepper, to taste

- 1/4 cup orange segments, for garnish

- Fresh mint leaves, for garnish

Directions:

1. Arrange the mixed salad greens on a large serving platter or divide among individual plates.

2. Top the greens with sliced roasted beets, spreading them out evenly over the salad.

3. Sprinkle the toasted walnuts and crumbled goat cheese over the beets.

4. In a small bowl, whisk together the balsamic vinegar and olive oil. Season with salt and pepper to taste.

5. Drizzle the dressing over the salad just before serving.

6. Garnish with orange segments and fresh mint leaves.

Per serving: Calories: 320; Fat: 27g; Protein: 8g; Carbs: 15g; Sugar: 9g; Fiber: 4g

Difficulty rating: ★☆☆☆☆

Allergen information: Gluten-free, Nut-free.

---

105. Spinach and Strawberry Salad

Prep time: 15 minutes

Cook time: 0 minutes

Serves: 4

Ingredients:

- 4 cups baby spinach, washed and dried

- 1 cup strawberries, sliced

- 1/2 cup cucumber, thinly sliced

- 1/4 cup walnuts, chopped

- 1/4 cup feta cheese, crumbled (lactose-free if necessary)

- 2 tablespoons balsamic vinegar

- 1 tablespoon olive oil

- Salt and pepper, to taste

Preparation instructions:

1. In a large salad bowl, combine the baby spinach, sliced strawberries, and sliced cucumber.

2. Add the chopped walnuts and crumbled feta cheese to the salad.

3. In a small bowl, whisk together the balsamic vinegar and olive oil. Season with salt and pepper to taste.

4. After adding the dressing to the salad, gently mix to coat all of the ingredients.

5. Serve immediately, or chill in the refrigerator for up to an hour before serving.

Per serving: Calories: 180; Fat: 14g; Protein: 5g; Carbs: 10g; Sugar: 6g; Fiber: 2g

Difficulty rating: ★☆☆☆☆

Allergen information: Gluten-free, Nut-free option (omit walnuts), Dairy-free option (omit feta or use dairy-free cheese).

Desserts

Prep time: 10 minutes

Cook time: 0 minutes

Serves: 2

Ingredients:

- 1 cup silken tofu
- 1/4 cup cocoa powder
- 1/4 cup maple syrup
- 1/2 teaspoon vanilla extract
- Pinch of salt
- Fresh berries, for garnish
- Mint leaves, for garnish

Preparation instructions:

1. Place the silken tofu, cocoa powder, maple syrup, vanilla extract, and a pinch of salt in a blender or food processor.

2. Blend until creamy and smooth, stopping occasionally to scrape down the sides.

3. Divide the mousse between two serving dishes and refrigerate for at least 30 minutes to chill.

4. Garnish with fresh berries and mint leaves before serving.

Per serving: Calories: 180;Fat: 9g; Protein: 6g; Carbs: 28g; Sugar: 18g; Fiber: 4g

Difficulty rating: ★☆☆☆☆

Allergen information: Gluten-free, Dairy-free, Nut-free.

Prep time: 20 minutes

Cook time: 35 minutes

Serves: 12 bars

Ingredients:

- 1 1/2 cups almond flour
- 1/4 cup coconut oil, melted
- 2 tablespoons maple syrup
- 1 teaspoon vanilla extract
- 1/4 teaspoon salt
- 8 oz lactose-free cream cheese, softened
- 1/4 cup granulated sugar
- 1 large egg
- 1/2 teaspoon lemon zest
- 2 tablespoons lemon juice
- 1/2 cup blueberries

Directions:

1. Set the oven's temperature to 175°C/350°F. Using parchment paper, line an 8-inch square baking dish, leaving a small overhang for easy removal.

2. Almond flour, melted coconut oil, maple syrup, salt, and vanilla essence should all be combined in a bowl. Firmly press the mixture into the bottom of the baking dish that has been prepared.

3. After 10 minutes of baking, take the crust out of the oven and allow it to cool somewhat.

4. In a separate bowl, beat the lactose-free cream cheese and granulated sugar until smooth. Add the egg, lemon zest, and lemon juice, beating until well combined.

5. Pour the cream cheese mixture over the cooled crust and smooth the top with a spatula.

6. Scatter the blueberries evenly over the top of the cream cheese layer.

7. Bake for twenty-five minutes, or until the middle of the filling is firm but still jiggly.

8. Allow the bars to cool to room temperature, then refrigerate for at least 3 hours or overnight.

9. Before serving, remove the bars from the pan using the parchment paper overhang and cut them into 12 squares.

Per serving: Calories: 220; Fat: 18g; Protein: 5g; Carbs: 12g; Sugar: 8g; Fiber: 2g

Difficulty rating: ★★☆☆☆

Allergen information: Gluten-free, Dairy-free (lactose-free cream cheese).

---

108. Coconut Macaroons

Prep time: 15 minutes

Cook time: 15 minutes

Serves: 4

Ingredients:

- 2 cups unsweetened shredded coconut

- 3 tablespoons maple syrup

- 2 tablespoons coconut oil, melted

- 1/2 teaspoon vanilla extract

- 1/4 teaspoon salt

- 2 large egg whites

Preparation instructions:

1. Preheat the oven to 325°F (163°C), and place parchment paper on a baking pan.

2. Put the shredded coconut, salt, vanilla essence, melted coconut oil, and maple syrup in a big bowl. Until all the ingredients are well incorporated, mix well.

3. Beat the egg whites in a another dish until firm peaks form. Making sure not to deflate the egg whites, gently fold them into the coconut mixture until just incorporated.

4. Form the mixture into small mounds on the prepared baking sheet, about an inch apart, using a tablespoon or small cookie scoop.

5. Bake in the preheated oven for 12-15 minutes, or until the macaroons are golden around the edges.

6. After five minutes of cooling on the baking sheet, move the macaroons to a wire rack to finish cooling.

Per serving: Calories: 280; Fat: 20g; Protein: 3g; Carbs: 24g; Sugar: 18g; Fiber: 5g

Difficulty rating: ★☆☆☆☆

Allergen information: Gluten-free, Dairy-free.

---

109. Almond Flour Brownies

Prep time: 15 minutes

Cook time: 25 minutes

Serves: 8

Ingredients:

- 2 cups almond flour

- 1/4 cup cocoa powder

- 1/2 teaspoon baking soda

- 1/4 teaspoon salt

- 1/2 cup unsalted butter, melted

- 3/4 cup maple syrup

- 2 large eggs

- 1 teaspoon vanilla extract

- 1/2 cup dark chocolate chips (ensure dairy-free for a fully low-FODMAP diet)

Directions:

1. Preheat the oven to 350°F (175°C). Line an 8-inch square baking pan with parchment paper, leaving an overhang on the sides for easy removal.

2. In a medium bowl, whisk together almond flour, cocoa powder, baking soda, and salt.

3. Gently whisk together the eggs, maple syrup, vanilla extract, and melted butter in a large basin.

4. Stirring until just blended, gradually add the dry ingredients to the wet components. Add the dark chocolate chips and fold.

5. Pour the batter into the prepared baking pan, smoothing the top with a spatula.

6. Bake for 25 minutes, or until a toothpick inserted into the center comes out with a few moist crumbs.

7. Let the brownies cool completely in the pan set on a wire rack. Once cooled, use the parchment paper overhang to lift the brownies out of the pan and cut into squares.

Per serving: Calories: 320; Fat: 24g; Protein: 7g; Carbs: 23g; Sugar: 15g; Fiber: 4g

Difficulty rating: ★★☆☆☆

Allergen information: Gluten-free, Dairy-free option (use dairy-free chocolate chips).

---

110. Pumpkin Pie Bites

Prep time: 20 minutes

Cook time: 15 minutes

Serves: 12 bites

Ingredients:

- 1 cup canned pumpkin puree

- 1/4 cup almond flour

- 1/4 cup coconut flour

- 2 tablespoons maple syrup

- 1 teaspoon pumpkin pie spice

- 1/2 teaspoon vanilla extract

- Pinch of salt

- 1/4 cup dark chocolate chips, dairy-free

Preparation instructions:

1. Pumpkin puree, almond flour, coconut flour, maple syrup, pumpkin pie spice, vanilla essence, and a dash of salt should all be combined in a

sizable mixing dish. Mix thoroughly until a dough forms.

2. Fold in the dark chocolate chips.

3. Using a tablespoon, scoop the dough and roll into balls. Place the balls on a parchment-lined baking sheet.

4. Refrigerate the pumpkin pie bites for at least 1 hour to set.

5. Before serving, you can optionally melt additional dark chocolate and drizzle over the bites for extra decadence.

Per serving: Calories: 90; Fat: 4g; Protein: 2g; Carbs: 12g; Sugar: 6g; Fiber: 3g

Difficulty rating: ★☆☆☆☆

Allergen information: Gluten-free, Dairy-free.

---

111. Raspberry Chia Seed Pudding

Prep time: 10 minutes

Cook time: 0 minutes

Serves: 2

Ingredients:

- 1/4 cup chia seeds

- 1 cup unsweetened almond milk

- 1 tablespoon maple syrup

- 1/2 teaspoon vanilla extract

- 1/2 cup fresh raspberries

- Additional raspberries and mint leaves, for garnish

Preparation instructions:

1. In a bowl, combine the chia seeds, almond milk, maple syrup, and vanilla extract. Stir well to mix.

2. Gently fold in the fresh raspberries.

3. After the mixture thickens and the chia seeds have absorbed the liquid, cover the bowl and place it in the refrigerator for at least 4 hours, or overnight.

4. When the pudding sets, stir it to make sure the consistency is uniform. To get the right consistency, if the pudding is too thick, add a little extra almond milk.

5. Serve the pudding in bowls or glasses, garnished with additional raspberries and mint leaves.

Per serving: Calories: 180; Fat: 9g; Protein: 4g; Carbs: 23g; Sugar: 10g; Fiber: 10g

Difficulty rating: ★☆☆☆☆

Allergen information: Gluten-free, Dairy-free, Nut-free (note: ensure almond milk is suitable for those with nut allergies or substitute with a nut-free milk alternative).

112. Peanut Butter Cookies

Prep time: 15 minutes

Cook time: 12 minutes

Serves: 12 cookies

Ingredients:

- 1 cup natural peanut butter (smooth or crunchy)

- 3/4 cup granulated sugar

- 1 large egg

- 1 teaspoon baking soda

- 1/2 teaspoon vanilla extract

- Pinch of salt

- 1/4 cup dark chocolate chips (optional, ensure low-FODMAP friendly)

Directions:

1. Preheat the oven to 350°F (175°C) and line a baking sheet with parchment paper.

2. In a mixing bowl, combine the peanut butter, sugar, egg, baking soda, vanilla extract, and a pinch of salt. Stir well until the mixture is smooth and fully combined.

3. If using, fold in the dark chocolate chips.

4. Scoop tablespoon-sized amounts of the dough onto the prepared baking sheet, spacing them about 2 inches apart.

5. Using the back of a fork, gently flatten each dough ball to make a crossing design.

6. Bake in the preheated oven for 10-12 minutes, or until the edges are golden and the centers are set.

7. After five minutes of cooling on the baking sheet, move the cookies to a wire rack to finish cooling.

Per serving: Calories: 180; Fat: 12g; Protein: 6g; Carbs: 15g; Sugar: 13g; Fiber: 1g

Difficulty rating: ★☆☆☆☆

Allergen information: Gluten-free, Dairy-free (without chocolate chips or using dairy-free chips).

---

113. Pineapple Sorbet

Prep time: 10 minutes

Cook time: 0 minutes

Serves: 4

Ingredients:

- 3 cups ripe pineapple, chopped and frozen

- 1/4 cup maple syrup

- 1/2 cup coconut milk

- 1 tablespoon lime juice

Directions:

1. Place the frozen pineapple, maple syrup, coconut milk, and lime juice in a blender or food processor.

2. Blend until creamy and smooth, stopping occasionally to scrape down the sides.

3. To get the right consistency, if the mixture is too thick, add a bit extra coconut milk.

4. Once blended to a smooth sorbet texture, transfer the mixture to a freezer-safe container.

5. Freeze for at least 2 hours or until firm.

6. Allow the sorbet to soften slightly at room temperature for a few minutes before serving.

7. Serve in bowls or dessert glasses, garnished with fresh pineapple pieces or lime zest, if desired.

Per serving: Calories: 150; Fat: 3g; Protein: 1g; Carbs: 32g; Sugar: 28g; Fiber: 2g

Difficulty rating: ★☆☆☆☆

Allergen information: Gluten-free, Dairy-free, Nut-free

---

114. Cinnamon Banana Crisp

Prep time: 15 minutes

Cook time: 45 minutes

Serves: 6

Ingredients:

- 4 cups diced firm, unripe bananas

- 1 tablespoon lemon juice

- 1/2 cup granulated sugar

- 1 teaspoon ground cinnamon

- 1/4 teaspoon ground nutmeg

- 1 cup gluten-free rolled oats

- 1/2 cup almond flour

- 1/2 cup brown sugar, packed

- 1/4 teaspoon salt

- 6 tablespoons unsalted butter, melted

- 1/2 teaspoon vanilla extract

Preparation instructions:

1. Preheat the oven to 350°F (175°C). Grease an 8-inch square baking dish with butter or non-stick spray.

2. Diced bananas should be nicely covered after being tossed in a big basin with ground nutmeg, ground cinnamon, granulated sugar, and lemon juice. Spread the banana mixture equally in the baking dish that has been prepared.

3. In the same bowl, combine the gluten-free rolled oats, almond flour, brown sugar, and salt. Pour in the melted butter and vanilla extract, and mix until the dry ingredients are moistened and the mixture clumps together.

4. Sprinkle the oat mixture evenly over the bananas in the baking dish.

5. Bake in the preheated oven for 45 minutes, or until the topping is golden brown and the bananas are tender when pierced with a fork.

6. Allow the crisp to cool slightly before serving. It can be served warm or at room temperature.

Per serving: Calories: 350; Fat: 16g; Protein: 4g; Carbs: 50g; Sugar: 38g; Fiber: 4g

Difficulty rating: ★☆☆☆☆

Allergen information: Gluten-free, Nut-free (Note: Almond flour is used, please ensure no nut allergies before serving).

Prep time: 15 minutes

Cook time: 5 minutes

Serves: 4

Ingredients:

- 2 cups lactose-free milk or almond milk

- 1 tablespoon gelatin powder

- 3 tablespoons maple syrup

- 1 teaspoon vanilla extract

- 1/2 cup fresh berries for topping

- Mint leaves for garnish (optional)

Preparation instructions:

1. Pour 1/2 cup of the lactose-free milk or almond milk into a small bowl. Sprinkle the gelatin powder over the milk and let it sit for about 5 minutes to soften.

2. The leftover 1 1/2 cups of milk should be heated in a saucepan over medium heat. Avoid boiling. When the milk is warm, add the softened gelatin mixture and whisk until the gelatin is completely dissolved.

3. After turning off the heat, add the vanilla extract and maple syrup to the pot.

4. Divide the mixture evenly among four serving glasses or ramekins. Refrigerate for at least 4 hours, or until set.

5. Before serving, top each panna cotta with fresh berries and garnish with mint leaves if desired.

Per serving: Calories: 120; Fat: 2g; Protein: 4g; Carbs: 20g; Sugar: 16g; Fiber: 1g

Difficulty rating: ★☆☆☆☆

Allergen information: Gluten-free, Dairy-free (if using almond milk).

Prep time: 20 minutes

Cook time: 15 minutes

Serves: 4

Ingredients:

- 2 cups gluten-free all-purpose flour

- 1/4 cup granulated sugar

- 1 tablespoon baking powder

- 1/2 teaspoon salt

- 3/4 cup lactose-free milk

- 1/4 cup unsalted butter, melted

- 1 large egg

- 1 teaspoon vanilla extract

- 1 cup fresh strawberries, diced

- 1/2 cup whipped cream (lactose-free if necessary)

Directions:

1. Preheat the oven to 425°F (220°C). Line a baking sheet with parchment paper.

2. In a large bowl, whisk together the gluten-free flour, granulated sugar, baking powder, and salt.

3. In a separate bowl, mix the lactose-free milk, melted butter, egg, and vanilla extract until well combined.

4. Gradually add the wet ingredients to the dry ingredients, stirring until just combined. Do not overmix.

5. Gently fold in the diced strawberries.

6. Using spoons, drop batter onto the baking sheet that has been prepared to produce 8 shortcakes.

7. Bake for 15 minutes, or until a toothpick inserted in the center comes out clean and the shortcakes are brown.

8. Let the shortcakes cool a little bit on the baking sheet, then move them to a wire rack to finish cooling.

9. To serve, split each shortcake in half horizontally. Spoon whipped cream and additional fresh strawberries between the layers and on top.

Per serving: Calories: 350; Fat: 12g; Protein: 6g; Carbs: 56g; Sugar: 18g; Fiber: 3g

Difficulty rating: ★★☆☆☆

Allergen information: Gluten-free, Nut-free.

---

117. Banana Oatmeal Cookies

Prep time: 15 minutes

Cook time: 12 minutes

Serves: 12 cookies

Ingredients:

- 2 small ripe bananas, mashed (use just-ripe, firm bananas to stay within low-FODMAP limits)

- 1 cup gluten-free rolled oats

- 1/2 cup dark chocolate chips (choose low-FODMAP certified or limit to 20g per serving)

- 1/4 cup walnuts, chopped (optional, limit to 10 halves per serving if included)

- 1 tsp vanilla extract

- 1/2 tsp cinnamon

- A pinch of salt

Preparation instructions:

1. Preheat your oven to 350°F (175°C) and line a baking sheet with parchment paper.

2. In a large bowl, combine the mashed bananas with the gluten-free rolled oats, dark chocolate chips, chopped walnuts (if using), vanilla extract, cinnamon, and a pinch of salt. Mix until well combined.

3. Drop spoonfuls of the cookie dough onto the lined baking sheet to create 12 uniformly sized cookies. Using the back of the spoon, slightly flatten each dollop.

4. Bake in the preheated oven for 12 minutes, or until the edges of the cookies are golden brown.

5. Take the cookies out of the oven and allow them to rest for five minutes on the baking sheet before moving them to a wire rack to cool down fully.

Per serving: Calories: 90; Fat: 3g; Protein: 2g; Carbs: 15g; Sugar: 6g; Fiber: 2g

Difficulty rating: ★☆☆☆☆

Allergen information: Gluten-free, Dairy-free, Nut-free option (omit walnuts).

---

118. Blueberry Lemon Muffins

Prep time: 15 minutes

Cook time: 25 minutes

Serves: 12

Ingredients:

- 2 cups gluten-free all-purpose flour

- 1/2 cup granulated sugar

- 2 teaspoons baking powder

- 1/2 teaspoon baking soda

- 1/4 teaspoon salt

- 3/4 cup lactose-free milk

- 1/3 cup vegetable oil

- 1 large egg

- 1 tablespoon lemon zest

- 1/4 cup fresh lemon juice

- 1 cup fresh blueberries

Directions:

1. Turn the oven on to 375°F, or 190°C. Use paper liners or non-stick cooking spray to coat a muffin pan.

2. In a large mixing bowl, whisk together the gluten-free flour, sugar, baking powder, baking soda, and salt.

3. In a separate bowl, mix the lactose-free milk, vegetable oil, egg, lemon zest, and lemon juice until well combined.

4. Add the liquid mixture to the dry mixture and whisk just until blended. Fold in the blueberries gently.

5. Evenly distribute the batter into each muffin cup, filling them to about two-thirds of the way.

6. Bake the muffins for twenty-five minutes, or until a toothpick inserted into the center of one comes out clean.

7. Let the muffins cool in the pan for 5 minutes before transferring to a wire rack to cool completely.

Per serving: Calories: 190; Fat: 7g; Protein: 3g; Carbs: 30g; Sugar: 12g; Fiber: 1g

Difficulty rating: ★☆☆☆☆

Allergen information: Gluten-free, Dairy-free

Prep time: 15 minutes

Cook time: 55 minutes

Serves: 8

Ingredients:

- 2 cups gluten-free all-purpose flour

- 1 teaspoon baking soda

- 1/4 teaspoon salt

- 4 ripe bananas, mashed

- 1/2 cup sugar

- 1/2 cup brown sugar, packed

- 1/2 cup unsalted butter, melted and cooled (use lactose-free if necessary)

- 2 large eggs, beaten

- 1/4 cup lactose-free milk

- 1 teaspoon vanilla extract

- 1 cup dark chocolate chips (ensure dairy-free if necessary)

Directions:

1. Preheat the oven to 350°F (175°C). Grease a 9x5 inch loaf pan and set aside.

2. In a large bowl, whisk together the gluten-free flour, baking soda, and salt.

3. In another bowl, mix the mashed bananas with sugar, brown sugar, melted butter, eggs, lactose-free milk, and vanilla extract until well combined.

4. Stirring until just blended, gradually add the dry ingredients to the wet components. Add the chocolate chips and fold.

5. Transfer the batter into the loaf pan that has been ready and use a spatula to level the top.

6. Bake for 55 minutes, or until a toothpick inserted in the center comes out clean, in a preheated oven.

7. Allow the bread to cool in the pan for 10 minutes, then transfer to a wire rack to cool completely before slicing.

Per serving: Calories: 420; Fat: 19g; Protein: 5g; Carbs: 62g; Sugar: 35g; Fiber: 4g

Difficulty rating: ★★☆☆☆

Allergen information: Gluten-free, Dairy-free option (use dairy-free butter and chocolate chips), Nut-free.

120. Coconut Lime Bars

Prep time: 20 minutes

Cook time: 15 minutes

Serves: 12 bars

Ingredients:

- 1 1/2 cups almond flour

- 1/4 cup coconut oil, melted

- 2 tablespoons maple syrup

- 1/4 teaspoon salt

- 1 cup unsweetened shredded coconut

- 1/2 cup lime juice (about 4 limes)

- 1/2 cup canned coconut milk

- 1/3 cup maple syrup

- 4 large eggs

- 1 tablespoon lime zest

- 1/4 cup almond flour

Directions:

1. Set the oven's temperature to 175°C/350°F. Using parchment paper, line an 8 by 8-inch baking pan, leaving an overhang for easy removal from the sides.

2. In a medium bowl, combine 1 1/2 cups almond flour, melted coconut oil, 2 tablespoons maple syrup, and salt. Press the mixture firmly into the bottom of the prepared pan. Bake for 10 minutes, then remove from the oven and let cool slightly.

3. In a large bowl, whisk together the shredded coconut, lime juice, coconut milk, 1/3 cup maple syrup, eggs, and lime zest until well combined. Stir in 1/4 cup almond flour.

4. Pour the lime and coconut mixture over the cooled crust. Return to the oven and bake for an additional 15 minutes, or until the filling is set.

5. Allow the bars to cool fully on a wire rack within the pan. After the bars have cooled, remove them from the pan by using the overhanging parchment paper. Divide into twelve bars.

6. Before serving, let the bars cool in the fridge for at least two hours. Any leftovers should be refrigerated in an airtight container.

Per serving: Calories: 230; Fat: 17g; Protein: 5g; Carbs: 16g; Sugar: 9g; Fiber: 3g

Difficulty rating: ★★☆☆☆

Allergen information: Gluten-free, Dairy-free.

60-Day Meal Plan

First 30-Day Plan

Day	Breakfast	Lunch	Dinner	Snack
1	Blueberry Almond Overnight Oats	Grilled Chicken Caesar Salad	Citrus Herb Grilled Chicken	Baked Sweet Potato Fries
2	Spinach and Feta Omelette	Turkey and Swiss Sandwich	Baked Cod with Dill	Golden Zucchini Bites
3	Banana Walnut Pancakes	Quinoa and Roasted Vegetable Bowl	Herb-Crusted Chicken with Roasted Vegetables	Carrot and Ginger Soup
4	Quinoa Breakfast Bowl	Chicken Herb Salad with Lemon Vinaigrette	Quinoa Stuffed Bell Peppers	Shrimp with Pineapple Salsa
5	Chia Seed Pudding with Berries	Lentil and Spinach Soup	Lemon Shrimp Skewers	Zucchini Hummus and Veggie Platter
6	Sweet Potato Hash with Eggs	Tuna Salad Lettuce Wraps	Beef and Vegetable Stir-Fry	Turkey and Cream Cheese Roll-Ups
7	Greek Yogurt Parfait	Vegetable and Hummus Wrap	Chicken and Broccoli Casserole	Cottage Cheese and Pineapple Bowl
8	Avocado and Egg Toast	Chicken and Rice Soup	Turkey Meatballs with Zucchini Noodles	Rice Paper Veggie Rolls
9	Gluten-Free Waffles	Mediterranean Veggie Salad	Salmon with Zucchini and Lemon Dill	Baked Vegetable Egg Muffins
10	Pumpkin Spice Smoothie	Beef and Broccoli Delight	Vegetable Paella	Chicken and Veggie Lettuce Boats
11	Coconut Flour Muffins	Shrimp and Quinoa Salad	Herb-Roasted Pork and Vegetables	Cucumber and Dill Salad
12	Scrambled Tofu with Vegetables	Egg Salad Sandwich	Lentil and Vegetable Stew	Baked Sweet Potato Fries
13	Buckwheat Porridge	Roasted Vegetable and Goat Cheese Salad	Chicken Fajita Bowls	Turkey and Cream Cheese Roll-Ups
14	Blueberry Cinnamon Breakfast Bars	Chicken and Zucchini Noodles	Spaghetti Squash with Marinara	Shrimp with Pineapple Salsa

Day	Breakfast	Lunch	Dinner	Snack
15	Smoked Salmon and Cream Cheese Bagel	Turkey Chili	Tofu and Vegetable Stir-Fry	Carrot and Ginger Soup
16	Pumpkin Spice Smoothie	Turkey and Swiss Sandwich	Lemon Herb Chicken Thighs	Baked Sweet Potato Fries
17	Coconut Flour Muffins	Quinoa and Roasted Vegetable Bowl	Baked Lemon Butter Tilapia	Golden Zucchini Bites
18	Buckwheat Porridge	Chicken Herb Salad with Lemon Vinaigrette	Butter Shrimp Scampi	Carrot and Ginger Soup
19	Blueberry Cinnamon Breakfast Bars	Lentil and Spinach Soup	Cajun Blackened Catfish	Shrimp with Pineapple Salsa
20	Smoked Salmon and Cream Cheese Bagel	Tuna Salad Lettuce Wraps	Maple-Ginger Lemon Salmon	Zucchini Hummus and Veggie Platter
21	Chia Seed Pudding with Berries	Vegetable and Hummus Wrap	Spicy Tuna Poke Bowl	Turkey and Cream Cheese Roll-Ups
22	Sweet Potato Hash with Eggs	Chicken and Rice Soup	Tropical Coconut Shrimp Delight	Cottage Cheese and Pineapple Bowl
23	Greek Yogurt Parfait	Mediterranean Veggie Salad	Pan-Seared Scallops with Lemon Herb Sauce	Rice Paper Veggie Rolls
24	Avocado and Egg Toast	Beef and Broccoli Delight	Baked Halibut with Tomato Basil Sauce	Baked Vegetable Egg Muffins
25	Gluten-Free Waffles	Shrimp and Quinoa Salad	Grilled Swordfish with Chimichurri	Chicken and Veggie Lettuce Boats
26	Banana Walnut Pancakes	Egg Salad Sandwich	Shrimp and Cucumber Salad	Cucumber and Dill Salad
27	Blueberry Almond Overnight Oats	Roasted Vegetable and Goat Cheese Salad	Lemon Dill Baked Cod	Baked Sweet Potato Fries
28	Spinach and Feta Omelette	Chicken and Zucchini Noodles	Herb-Crusted Lamb Chops	Turkey and Cream Cheese Roll-Ups
29	Quinoa Breakfast Bowl	Turkey Chili	Rosemary Pork Chops	Shrimp with Pineapple Salsa
30	Chia Seed Pudding with Berries	Chicken Herb Salad with Lemon Vinaigrette	Maple Mustard Baked Chicken Breasts	Carrot and Ginger Soup

Second 30-Day Plan

Day	Breakfast	Lunch	Dinner	Snacks
1	Smoked Salmon and Cream Cheese Bagel	Mexican Quinoa and Bean Salad	Herb-Crusted Chicken with Roasted Veggies	Hummus and Veggie Platter
2	Blueberry Cinnamon Breakfast Bars	Vegetable and Hummus Wrap	Beef and Mushroom Stroganoff	Rice Paper Veggie Rolls
3	Chia Seed Pudding with Berries	Grilled Chicken Caesar Salad	Maple-Ginger Lemon Salmon	Cottage Cheese and Pineapple Bowl
4	Sweet Potato Hash with Eggs	Chicken and Zucchini Noodles	Quinoa Stuffed Bell Peppers	Turkey and Cream Cheese Roll-Ups
5	Banana Walnut Pancakes	Mediterranean Chickpea Salad	Balsamic Glazed Pork Tenderloin	Baked Sweet Potato Fries
6	Quinoa Breakfast Bowl	Shrimp and Quinoa Salad	Rosemary Pork Chops	Golden Zucchini Bites
7	Gluten-Free Waffles	Beef and Broccoli Delight	Chicken and Broccoli Casserole	Cucumber and Dill Salad
8	Pumpkin Spice Smoothie	Lemon Chicken Orzo Soup	Turkey Meatballs with Zucchini Noodles	Carrot and Ginger Soup
9	Scrambled Tofu with Vegetables	Turkey Chili	Lemon Shrimp Skewers	Shrimp and Mango Salsa
10	Avocado and Egg Toast	Grilled Mahi Mahi with Pineapple Salsa	Citrus Herb Grilled Chicken	Lactose-Free Greek Yogurt with Strawberries
11	Buckwheat Porridge	Chicken and Avocado Salad	Stuffed Chicken Breasts with Spinach and Feta	Peanut Butter Cookies
12	Greek Yogurt Parfait	Egg Salad Sandwich	Lemon Dill Baked Cod	Pumpkin Pie Bites
13	Coconut Flour Muffins	Vegetarian Chili	Teriyaki Chicken Skewers	Almond Flour Brownies
14	Spinach and Feta Omelette	Chicken and Rice Soup	Cajun Spiced Chicken Wings	Coconut Macaroons
15	Blueberry Almond Overnight Oats	Lentil and Spinach Soup	Rosemary Roast Beef	Lemon Blueberry Cheesecake Bars
16	Spinach and Feta Omelette	Vegetarian Shepherd's Pie	Herb-Crusted Lamb Chops	Blueberry Lemon Muffins

Day	Breakfast	Lunch	Dinner	Snacks
17	Banana Walnut Pancakes	Quick & Easy Pad Thai	BBQ Pulled Pork	Banana Oatmeal Cookies
18	Pumpkin Spice Smoothie	Turkey and Swiss Sandwich	Salmon with Zucchini and Lemon Dill	Chocolate Mousse
19	Chia Seed Pudding with Berries	Quinoa and Roasted Vegetable Bowl	Grilled Swordfish with Chimichurri	Strawberry Shortcake
20	Sweet Potato Hash with Eggs	Tuna Salad Lettuce Wraps	Spaghetti Squash with Marinara	Raspberry Chia Seed Pudding
21	Quinoa Breakfast Bowl	Roasted Vegetable and Goat Cheese Salad	Tofu and Vegetable Stir-Fry	Vanilla Panna Cotta
22	Greek Yogurt Parfait	Chicken Fajita Bowls	Vegetarian Chili	Tropical Coconut Shrimp Delight
23	Scrambled Tofu with Vegetables	Vegetable Paella	Vegetarian Sushi Rolls	Spinach and Strawberry Salad
24	Pumpkin Spice Smoothie	Stuffed Zucchini Boats	Vegan Chickpea Curry	Cantaloupe and Feta Salad
25	Coconut Flour Muffins	Vegetarian Lasagna	Shrimp and Avocado Salad	Rustic Beet and Cheese Salad
26	Avocado and Egg Toast	Baked Cod with Dill	Vegetarian Shepherd's Pie	Asian Cabbage Salad
27	Gluten-Free Waffles	Shrimp and Mango Salsa	Vegan Stuffed Mushrooms	Kale and Quinoa Salad
28	Buckwheat Porridge	Grilled Vegetable Skewers	Maple Mustard Baked Chicken Breasts	Sweet and Savory Energy Balls
29	Blueberry Cinnamon Breakfast Bars	Roasted Red Pepper Soup	Vegetarian Pad Thai	Caprese Skewers
30	Spinach and Feta Omelette	Thai Coconut Shrimp Soup	Vegetable Paella	Cucumber Bites with Herb Cream Cheese

Conversion Tables

Accurate measurements are essential in maintaining the integrity of recipes, especially when managing a Low-FODMAP diet. These conversion tables are designed to help you seamlessly switch between different measurement systems, ensuring your culinary creations are both delicious and compliant with dietary needs.

Volume to weight conversions vary by ingredient due to differences in density. For example, a cup of strawberries weighs significantly less than a cup of sugar. These conversions are particularly crucial in baking, where precision can affect the texture and outcome of your dish.

Temperature conversions are also vital. Recipes often list temperatures in Fahrenheit or Celsius, and understanding these conversions ensures that dishes like Lemon Herb Chicken or Almond Flour Brownies are cooked perfectly every time.

Liquid measurements, especially between the U.S. system and the metric system, are essential for maintaining the balance of flavors. Knowing that 1 cup equals approximately 237 milliliters, or that 1 tablespoon is about 15 milliliters, can help you accurately follow recipes and avoid common pitfalls.

Lastly, converting gas mark settings to Fahrenheit or Celsius can save you from over or undercooking your food. With gas mark conversions readily available, you can confidently set your oven for recipes regardless of the original temperature notation.

By incorporating these tables, you can approach cooking with greater confidence and precision, ensuring that every meal supports your journey towards better digestive health.

Volume to Weight Conversions

Ingredient	Volume	Weight (grams)	Weight (ounces)
Sliced Strawberries	1 cup	152 g	5.4 oz
Sugar	1 cup	200 g	7 oz
Flour	1 cup	120 g	4.2 oz
Butter	1 cup	227 g	8 oz

Temperature Conversions

Temperature	Fahrenheit (°F)	Celsius (°C)
Boiling	212°F	100°C
Simmering	190-210°F	88-99°C
Baking	350°F	177°C
Freezing	32°F	0°C

Common Temperature Conversions

Gas Mark	Fahrenheit (°F)	Celsius (°C)
1	275°F	135°C
2	300°F	149°C
3	325°F	163°C
4	350°F	177°C
5	375°F	191°C
6	400°F	204°C
7	425°F	218°C

Liquid Measurements

Volume	U.S. (Cups)	Metric (Milliliters)
1 teaspoon (tsp)	1 tsp	5 ml
1 tablespoon (tbsp)	1 tbsp	15 ml
1/4 cup	0.25 cups	60 ml
1/3 cup	0.33 cups	80 ml
1/2 cup	0.5 cups	120 ml
1 cup	1 cup	237 ml
1 pint	2 cups	473 ml
1 quart	4 cups	946 ml
1 gallon	16 cups	3785 ml

Conclusion

Embarking on the Low-FODMAP journey marks the beginning of a transformative path toward improved digestive health and overall well-being. This cookbook has been crafted as a comprehensive guide to navigating the complexities of IBS and the dietary strategies that can alleviate its symptoms. Through the careful selection of ingredients and the preparation of the 120 recipes provided, individuals have the tools to experiment with a variety of dishes that not only cater to their dietary needs but also delight their palates.

The journey with IBS is deeply personal and varies from one individual to another, highlighting the importance of patience, experimentation, and adaptation. The initial phases of the diet, focusing on elimination and reintroduction, serve as foundational steps in understanding one's unique triggers and tolerances. It is through this process that one can tailor their diet to manage symptoms effectively while ensuring nutritional balance and enjoyment in eating.

The Low-FODMAP diet is not about restriction but about discovery—discovery of the foods that nourish and do not harm, of new recipes that bring joy to the kitchen and the table, and of the strength within to manage IBS with confidence and positivity. It encourages a proactive approach to health, advocating for informed choices, regular monitoring of symptoms, and engagement with healthcare professionals when needed.

As this journey unfolds, it becomes evident that managing IBS with a Low-FODMAP diet is a dynamic process, requiring ongoing adjustment and learning. This cookbook aims to be a trusted companion along the way, offering not just recipes but also a framework for living well with IBS. It is a testament to the resilience of those who navigate this path and a reminder of the vibrant life that awaits beyond IBS.

Remember, the path to better digestive health is paved with knowledge, support, and the delicious meals that have been shared in these pages. Here's to finding your balance, enjoying your meals, and embracing the journey ahead with optimism and grace.

★★★★★

With all my heart, I hope this book—which I put a lot of effort into writing—speaks to you. If the experience has been enjoyable for you, please think about giving an Amazon review. Your comments are helpful to me and to others who may not be aware of this work.

Scan here to submit a review

Recipe Index

Pumpkin Pie Bites; 92

Pumpkin Spice Smoothie; 21

Quinoa and Roasted Vegetable Bowl; 34

Quinoa Breakfast Bowl; 17

Quinoa Stuffed Bell Peppers; 45

Raspberry Chia Seed Pudding; 93

Rice Paper Veggie Rolls; 32

Roasted Red Pepper Soup; 83

Roasted Vegetable and Goat Cheese Salad; 41

Rosemary Roast Beef; 79

Rustic Beet and Cheese Salad; 88

Salmon with Zucchini and Lemon Dill; 48

Scrambled Tofu with Vegetables; 23

Shrimp and Avocado Salad; 72

Shrimp and Mango Salsa; 31

Shrimp and Quinoa Salad; 39

Smoked Salmon and Cream Cheese Bagel; 25

Spaghetti Squash with Marinara; 53

Spicy Beef Tacos; 76

Spicy Tuna Poke Bowl; 69

Spinach and Feta Omelette; 16

Spinach and Strawberry Salad; 89

Strawberry Shortcake; 96

Stuffed Chicken Breasts with Spinach and Feta; 81

Stuffed Zucchini Boats; 56

Sweet Potato Hash with Eggs; 19

Teriyaki Chicken Skewers; 77

Thai Coconut Shrimp Soup; 84

Tofu and Vegetable Stir-Fry; 54

Tropical Coconut Shrimp Delight; 70

Tuna Salad Lettuce Wraps; 36

Turkey and Cream Cheese Roll-Ups; 28

Turkey and Swiss Sandwich; 33

Turkey Chili; 42

Turkey Meatballs with Zucchini Noodles; 48

Vanilla Panna Cotta; 96

Vegan Black Bean Burgers; 61

Vegan Buddha Bowl; 58

Vegan Chickpea Curry; 65

Vegan Lentil Tacos; 55

Vegan Quinoa Salad; 59

Vegan Stuffed Mushrooms; 62

Vegetable and Hummus Wrap; 37

Vegetable Paella; 49

Vegetarian Chili; 57

Vegetarian Lasagna; 63

Vegetarian Pad Thai; 61

Vegetarian Shepherd's Pie; 64

Vegetarian Stuffed Peppers; 58

Vegetarian Sushi Rolls; 60

Zucchini and Turkey Roll-Ups; 29

Printed in Great Britain
by Amazon